The FITNESS CHALLENGE

RESHAPING OUR FUTURE

Rick C. Mason, Ph.D.

ISBN: 0985670622
ISBN-13: 987-0985670627

Big Picture Publishing

DEDICATION

To my family: Patty, Richard, and Ilene. Without them and their support, nothing in my life would be possible.

CONTENTS

ACKNOWLEDGMENTS

Special thanks go to Richard Mason for being my primary proofreader and sounding board.

Books by Rick C. Mason

The Big Picture: Life, Meaning, & Human Potential

INTRODUCTION

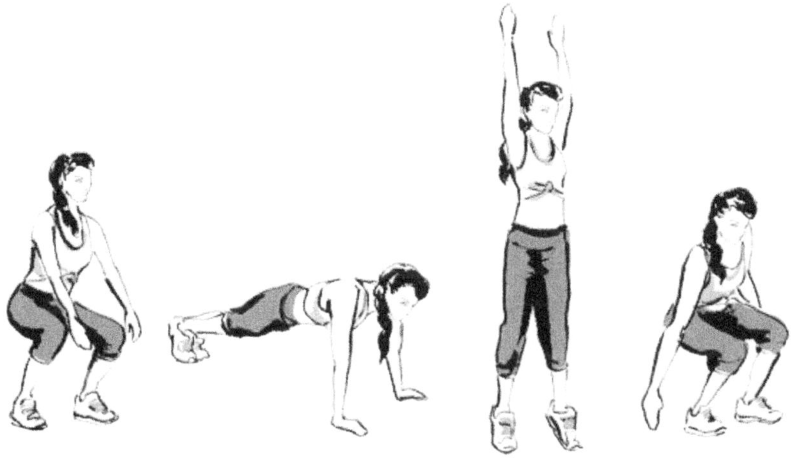

There is more wisdom in your body than in your deepest philosophy.
– Friedrich Nietzsche

As you probably already know, becoming fit is a major challenge, and only becoming more so, especially considering the environment in which we live today. Our postmodern world and lifestyle are working against us. Consider the following aspects of the world we currently occupy:

- We are surrounded by food, and much of it is easy to get and prepare.
- Much of the food that we have access to is highly processed and not good for us.
- We eat out much more often than we used to, and meals eaten at

restaurants tend to be higher in calories than those consumed at home.

- Unhealthy foods are less expensive than healthy ones.
- We are bombarded with advertisements encouraging us to eat and drink.
- We have machines that do our work for us.
- Most of us have jobs that require little physical work.
- Technology, like TV and computers, occupy an increasing amount of our time and keep us from moving.
- Physical education in many schools is either inadequate or has been cut due to lack of finances. Even school recess time – play time – has been reduced over recent decades.
- In the U.S., especially, it's difficult to ride a bike in most places. Walking is also difficult, or risky, in many urban areas due to poor planning and lack of sidewalks.

These conditions exert a cumulative effect over time, and, as a result, pose a danger to our individual and collective health. We keep getting fatter and less fit. Even for those with enough self-discipline to lose weight, most end up gaining it back. Our sorry state of fitness is contributing to disease and poor health. We are becoming weak, not only in terms of physical strength, but as a species as well. The explosion in the rate of obesity combined with a steep decline in levels of physical activity are morphing us into a new species of sorts – what I refer to as homo faticus. Our ancestors were lean and mean. They worked hard and were tough. I fear that if some catastrophe happened to cause us to revert back to the hard life they had, we would be so screwed.

The swift decline in our physical condition is only part of the problem. Healthcare costs associated with the treatment of obesity, diabetes, and related diseases threaten to bankrupt this country in the not-too-distant future. Right now obesity accounts for 21 percent of all health care costs, according to a study sponsored by Cornel University in 2012. This number is expected to rise in proportion with ballooning obesity rates. Obesity raises the costs of Medicaid, which means that we all pay for it through higher taxes.

Part of the problem is the speed in which obesity has overtaken us. Widespread obesity is a relatively recent development on the human timeline. Arising in the early-to-mid 20th century, it has taken obesity less than half a century to reach epidemic proportions in the developed world. In stark contrast to obesity, famine and starvation plagued humanity on a regular basis throughout history. Technological advances helped to create vast surpluses of food while simultaneously making our lives much less physically demanding. It seems as though we have become victims of our own prosperity. Too much food and too little exercise is a recipe for disaster, one that we are currently experiencing.

Our fitness continues to deteriorate, but it's not as if people aren't exposed to fitness concepts and opportunities. On the contrary, most people have access to well-equipped gyms or have exercise equipment in their home. In addition, there are a myriad of TV infomercials, books, magazines, and websites touting all kinds of diets, exercise equipment, and fitness programs. In short, we are deluged with messages extolling the virtues of fitness. So, what are we doing wrong? Why is fitness such a challenge? I'm actually referring to three distinct challenges:

1) The personal challenge of enhancing fitness
2) The challenge of maintaining high levels of fitness over a lifetime
3) The collective challenge facing our species to become more fit

The purpose of this book is to outline these challenges and to issue my own challenge to you. The bulk of this book details my own training and nutritional strategies, which have worked for me and can certainly work for you, too.

My first book, *The Big Picture*, detailed my philosophy of life, which states that our primary purpose in life is to strive actively for lifelong self-improvement. Fitness must be a major component of self-improvement. How can we function at our best and develop to our fullest potential unless we are healthy and physically fit? I believe that the importance of fitness in our lives cannot be overstated. Fitness, in fact, has such far reaching effects on our lives that it could rightly be considered a philosophy of life in itself. After all, the pursuit of fitness compels us to engage in health-promoting and character-building attitudes and behaviors. It also involves the setting of goals, dedication, will power, persistence, resolve, sacrifice, and other personal traits that are essential to the self-improvement process. Keeping with a "Big Picture" theme, a philosophy of fitness brings together these various aspects of fitness into a more unified and coherent picture.

I challenge you to use this book to develop your own philosophy of fitness. Consider my ideas and approaches critically, as you should for all information. My philosophy of fitness entails two major tenets that guide my thinking and behavior:

1) Fitness makes for a more productive and fulfilled life. Being fit enables one to take on life's challenges with vim and vigor.
2) Fitness contributes to a longer, healthier life and should be maintained over the lifespan.

I want to convince people that high levels of fitness can be achieved and maintained throughout our entire lifespan. I contend that by being more fit, most people could avoid many of the debilitating diseases we simply blame on the aging process.

There's now plenty of science informing us about the health benefits of regular exercise and sound nutrition, yet people are getting fatter and less fit. Far too many people don't exercise nearly enough. If we have any chance of reversing these dangerous trends, the pursuit of fitness must become a major component of our personal philosophy of life. We all must work toward cultivating a culture of fitness. In other words, fitness must become a personal lifestyle.

With this book, I present a complete philosophy of fitness. The word "philosophy" comes from the Greek meaning love of wisdom. Philosophy can be described as a system of beliefs, values, or tenets, as well as a personal outlook or viewpoint. One of the hallmarks of philosophy is its reliance on and promotion of critical thinking. Critical thinking requires us to question everything, including, and especially, our own thinking. For as long as I've been pursuing fitness, I continue to question my thinking and behaviors. Self-examination is critical to the self-improvement process. In developing my personal philosophy of fitness, I've integrated my past experiences with the latest scientific findings to identify specific tenets related to fitness.

You might be wondering if you really need a philosophy of fitness. After all, our knowledge of the human body, exercise, and nutrition increases almost daily. The problem is that most of this useful information goes unnoticed or is not applied in a meaningful way. People cling to outdated ideas and misinformation that keeps getting passed around. I want everyone to develop their own philosophy of fitness, but I want everyone to possess the best knowledge available. I want to change attitudes about fitness. It is important that people develop the attitude that the pursuit of fitness is much more than your diet and exercise routine; it's a total lifestyle.

Another important reason for me in writing this book is to promote the merits of critical thinking. Critical thinkers ask a lot of questions; they question their own assumptions; and they are able to weigh the merits of claims made by others through careful examination of evidence. With all my experience in the fitness arena, I can assure you that critical thinking is a vital component in the quest for fitness. Even the ancient Greeks advocated a proper balance between mind and body. Throughout history wise individuals have recognized the importance of developing the body and the mind. I am trying to maintain this health-promoting tradition. In fact, I argue that the body and mind are inseparable. You can't reach your full physical potential or utmost level of fitness without developing your mental prowess as well and vice versa. The pursuit of maximum fitness is a learning process, which requires one to commit to reading, observation, and critical thinking. And likewise, the active pursuit of fitness contributes to greater brain power, alleviation of stress, and higher levels of energy and positive mood, all of which sets the stage for enhanced learning.

Getting in shape and maintaining it over time is not easy. It doesn't help that there's so much conflicting information out there on how to train and how to eat. One must be able to think critically in order to make reasonable decisions concerning fitness. Many people waste considerable time and money trying everything under the sun. My primary goal with this book is to share my considerable knowledge and experience in the fitness arena so that you don't waste your time and money pursuing ineffective or inefficient fitness regimens. In addition, evidence concerning exercise and nutrition science is mounting and, in the process, is finally shattering many long-held myths.

In the chapters that follow I share with you my training and nutrition protocols, basically what I have learned through much trial and error and what I've found that works for me. But just as important, I want to equip you with the tools to think critically about your own approach to exercise and nutrition. Use this book as a guide only. Begin to think for yourself, in all areas, and don't believe everything you see and hear. Question what you read here. I want to make you think. Check the references I provide when I cite scientific studies. There is plenty of science to inform us on how to eat and exercise to attain our fitness potential. However, that doesn't necessarily mean that you will benefit fully from them. You might not like to eat the most nutritious foods, or you might not like to exercise at all. The most important thing is to engage in a fitness program or lifestyle that will help you improve but which is also something that you can live with and be happy.

To begin thinking critically about fitness, several important questions come to the fore. Many people simply take these questions for granted. We've been conditioned to think that we all need to do to become fit is to exercise regularly and eat healthy. But is this advice true for everyone? Here are what I believe to be important questions and ones that I address.

- What is fitness? What does it mean to be fit?
- Why is being fit important?
- To what lengths should we go in our pursuit of fitness?
- If exercise is so good for us, why don't more people exercise on a regular basis?
- How much exercise is enough, and what are the consequences, if any, of too much exercise?

Tenets of Fitness

To describe the tenets of fitness, I've created the acronym PLATES. "Plate" has several connections to fitness. Weight plates are the basic units of resistance training. We eat food off of plates, thus the nutrition angle. Finally, I like to compare the added muscle you'll have from lifting weights to armor plates, like those of a tank.

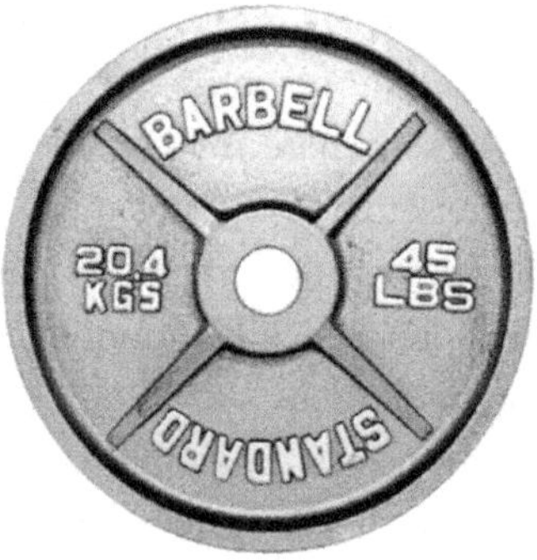

Priority: Fitness must be a priority. You must value it highly. You don't necessarily have to like exercise to place a value on fitness, but you must adopt behaviors that contribute to fitness.
Likeability: We tend to engage in activities that we like or are good at. Many people simply don't like structured exercise, but they may like to play

games that require movement. For the most part, do what you like. Just do something.

Accessibility: This is what we have access to in regard to fitness opportunities. Some can't afford a gym membership. Others may not have safe places to walk. Anyone can do jumping jacks in their living room, provided they have a living, or any, room.

Time: In today's hectic lifestyle, many people don't have time for a structured workout regimen. However, a structured regimen might not be necessary. Brief bursts of exercise, or activity, done often enough add up over time.

Efficiency: Total amount of work (exercise) completed in a given period of time. When time is limited, it becomes paramount to use it wisely. Therefore, it's generally better to do a high amount of work in a short period of time.

Safety: Which exercises can be done safely by an individual? Which foods should be avoided? This tenet involves the avoidance of injury and sickness. Injuries hinder your training goals and thus your pursuit of fitness.

Full Disclosure

Let me say right up front that I am not a medical doctor. None of my degrees are in a discipline directly related to fitness, health, or nutrition. My doctorate is in higher education policy. My expertise in the fitness arena comes from a lifetime of commitment to it. I've been going at this fitness thing, with a vengeance, for quite a while now. I have trained consistently for nearly 30 years, owned and operated a gym for 5 years, personally trained hundreds of people, and competed in bodybuilding, powerlifting, and half-marathon events. Moreover, I have read just about everything out there related to fitness.

I'll even admit to being addicted to exercise for the better part of my life, and may still be. Turning 50 has not slowed me down one bit, save a few more aches and pains. Maintaining a high level of fitness as an attempt to slow the aging process has become a personal challenge for me. I love a good challenge, and it is this persistent challenge of trying to improve that motivates me to keep working at it. However, getting older has imbued me with perspective. My enthusiasm for fitness is as strong as ever, but now I approach fitness in a more disciplined and mature manner.

My education has helped me become a more critical thinker. Achieving fitness requires much more than physical effort; it takes a good deal of mental effort as well. Sifting through all the information out there regarding fitness – much of it contradictory – requires critical thinking. You need to be prepared to evaluate claims and analyze arguments in order to make sound decisions regarding your personal fitness. It is my hope that this book will help you become more fit. To do so you will have to become a critical thinker. I challenge you to give it your best shot.

I must also advise you to get the okay from your doctor before beginning an exercise program. This is especially true if you are obese and/or have not exercised strenuously in a while. Intense exercise places stress on the body and in proportion to your body mass. You might have underlying health issues that could preclude you from engaging in intense exercise. So, get checked out, and if everything looks good and you are cleared to start exercising, begin slowly and gradually work your way up to higher levels of intensity. Remember that the goal is to adopt a fitness lifestyle, not to blindly pursue unrealistic expectations by trying to completely transform your body in just a few weeks.

1. WHAT IS FITNESS?

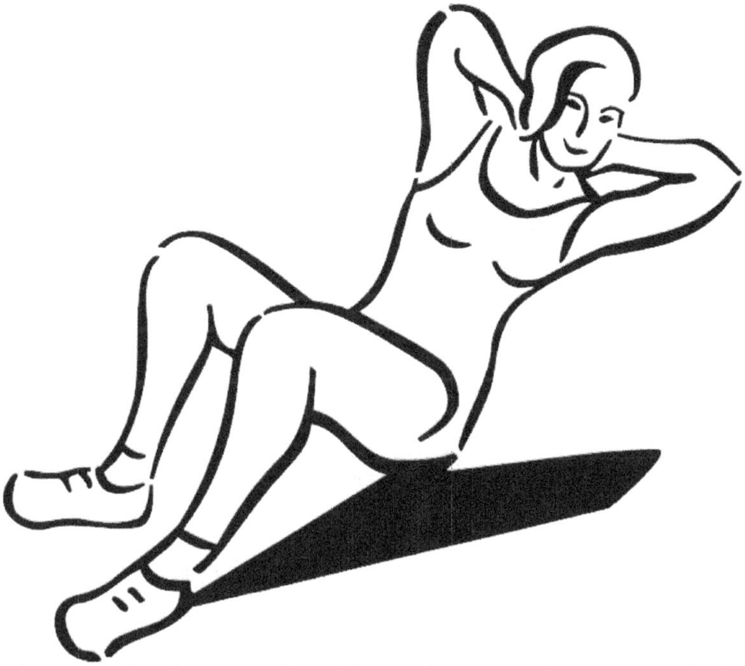

To keep the body in good health is a duty . . . otherwise we shall not be able to keep our mind strong and clear. – Buddha

In the past, "fitness" has been associated primarily with physical fitness. However, there's no doubt that physical fitness is closely related to overall health and well-being. So, to begin, I want to broaden what people think of when they think of fitness. Everyone wants to be more fit, but what does it mean to be fit? Is it how we feel? How we look? Our overall health? Traditionally, fitness has bordered on any or all of these things, but without sufficient specificity. When I use the term "fitness," I am referring to four broad, synergistic components of our lives, with each deserving significant attention:

- **Physique**: How our body looks. This often includes our level of bodyfat and muscle mass. A leaner, more muscular physique is generally considered more fit and aesthetically pleasing.

- **Conditioning**: How efficiently the body supplies blood and oxygen to working muscles, which dictates how long and hard we can work or exercise. Conditioning is enhanced primarily through aerobic exercise, like running, or weight training with lighter weight and higher reps with very little rest.
- **Well-Being**: How we feel, both physically and mentally. For most people, regular exercise enhances well-being, and individuals who report higher levels of well-being also report being happier and more productive.
- **Health**: Freedom from disease and sickness. Exercise and proper nutrition have been shown to enhance overall health. In general, improved fitness results in improved health.

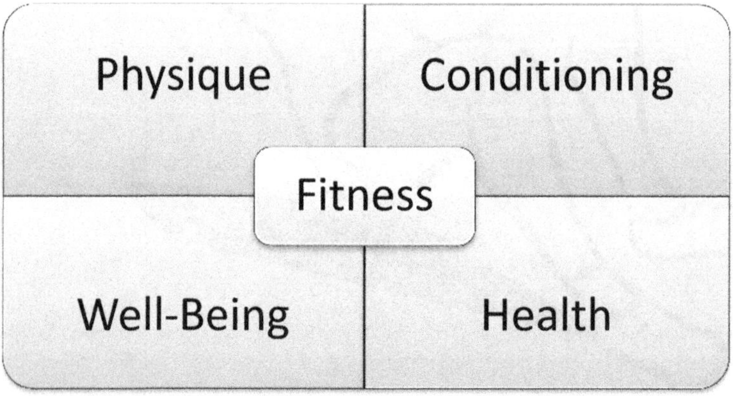

These components are closely related, in that each one is at least partly dependent upon the others. Fit people tend to be healthier, for instance. One could have a pleasing physique, however, and still be unhealthy or suffer from depression. Going in the other direction, there's plenty of overweight individuals who are remarkably healthy. So, even though each of these elements correlates positively with the others, it's far from perfect correlations. I want people to think and work more towards improving each of these facets of fitness.

Fitness describes a state of being whereby we maximize our individual potential in each of these areas. In the broader context, fitness is a lifestyle, which, at its core, involves all of the things one does on a regular basis to achieve and maintain a high degree of fitness. Small things done frequently and consistently can make a big difference by having a cumulative effect on the body.

Fitness also implies that we focus on what is true, or proven, in our fitness endeavors. There is so much misinformation out there, making it difficult to cut through the hype and outright lies. People need to know that they are not wasting their time, effort, and money on products and programs that will not produce (or have no chance of producing) the results that they so desperately desire. Those pursuing fitness seek to cut through the bologna and get to what has been proven to work.

We all want a better body. By "better," I mean that people, in general, want to look better, to have a more appealing physique. To most people, looking better means to be leaner with noticeable muscularity. People try to enhance their physiques for a number of reasons, but when you get to the heart of the matter, most people want to look better so they will be more attractive to potential mates. Nothing boosts our self-esteem more than the feeling of confidence that comes with enhancing our appearance. It's not all about aesthetics, though. Most men want to be bigger, since physical size in males is associated with higher status. In this respect, bigger really is better. Women, on the other hand, generally want to be smaller, as they feel that men are attracted more to smaller women. Moreover, people who exercise regularly feel better about themselves; they also feel better physically, have more energy, and are, generally, healthier than those less active. In short, physical fitness translates into real-world benefits, not the least of which is increased life span.

Conditioning has to do with how efficient the body's systems are functioning, especially the cardiovascular system. The cardiovascular system provides every cell in our body with oxygen while simultaneously ridding the cells of carbon dioxide, which is expelled when we exhale. Individuals who have placed increased demands on their cardiovascular systems through hard work/exercise are able to work harder and longer. Conditioning is typically measured by how much work one can do in a given amount of time. Conditioning and "shape" are nearly synonymous. While there's quite a bit of overlap between the terms, shape leans more towards how one's body looks. "Wow! Look at how toned she is." "Yeah, she's in great shape." Condition implies function and/or performance. "Rory has a resting pulse rate of 45." "Yeah, he's in fantastic condition." To me, both terms equate to greater health, above average levels of strength and endurance for one's age, and having a lean, aesthetically-pleasing physique.

Well-being has to do with how we feel, which can entail several perspectives. Obviously, we feel bad when we are sick, but this is usually a temporary condition. What I am getting at with well-being is how we think and feel about ourselves, our self-esteem and/or general mood. Regular exercise has been shown to elevate both significantly, which could contribute greatly to positive life outcomes.

Health has to do with the proper functioning of the body's systems, freedom from disease or infection within the body, and having the energy and spirit to perform one's duties and avocations. There are accepted methods to determine the state of one's health, including blood and urine tests, blood pressure, and stress tests, as examples. Of course, body composition and condition are also related to one's health, but that's not to say that you can't be overweight and be healthy; you can, just the same way a lean person can be unhealthy. In many ways, "healthy" simply means normal or free from disease. "Wellness" connotes holistic well-being, including physical, psychological, and even spiritual health. Personal wellness involves a life balance, much like the mind/body duality advocated by the ancient Greeks.

Our Current Condition

With all the known health benefits associated with increased fitness and all the emphasis placed on it in our culture, you would think that our level of fitness would be improving. However, you would be dead wrong. In fact, most Americans are in bad shape, physically, and, according to most measures, only getting worse. There is good reason for alarm. Consider the following statistics which are well documented from several reputable sources:

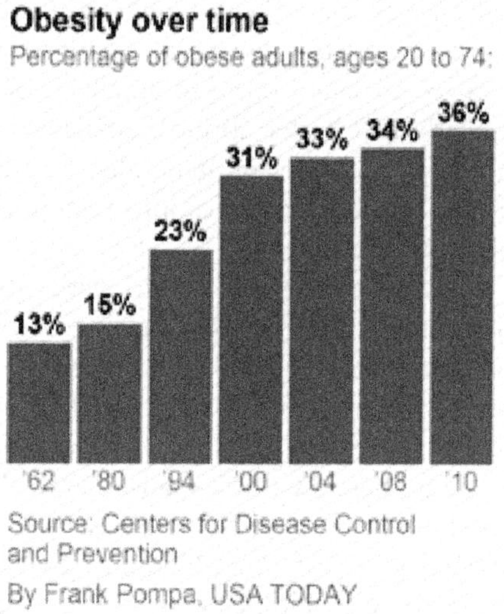

- More than two-thirds of adults are considered to be overweight or obese, and more than one-third are considered to be obese.
- About one-third of children/adolescents aged 6-19 are considered to be overweight or obese, and more than 1 in 6 are considered to be obese.
- The rate of obesity among adults has more than doubled since 1960, going from 13.4 to 35.7 percent.
- Adult obesity rates rose in 16 states during the past year and declined in none.
- 12 states, centered in the southeast, have obesity rates that exceed 30 percent.

- Just 10 years ago, no state had an obesity rate over 24 percent.
- The U.S. now leads the world in the rate of obesity.

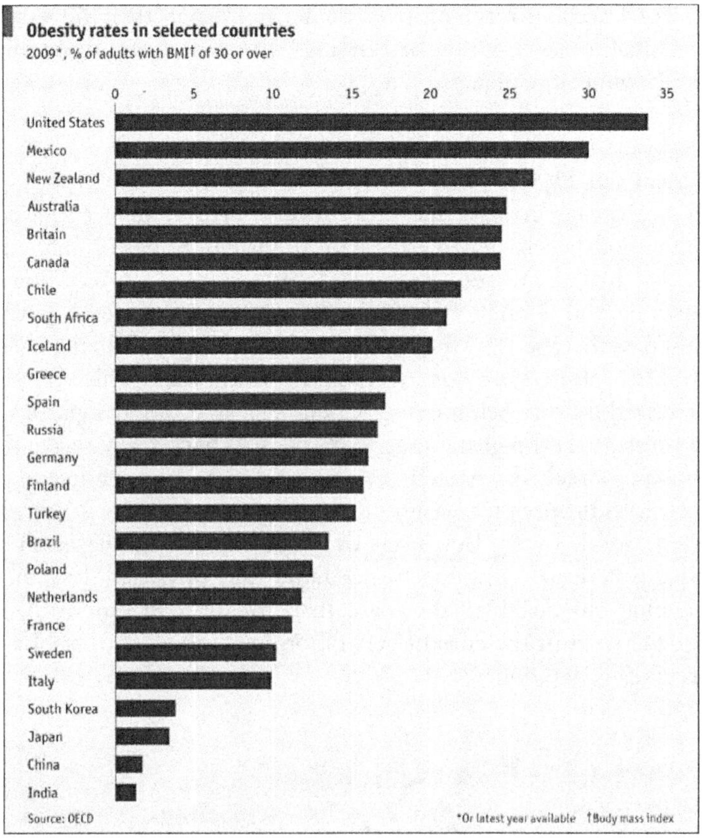

- In 8 states, more than 10 percent of adults now have type-II diabetes.
- Over the past 15 years, the rate of diabetes has doubled in 10 states.
- Only 49 percent of boys (age 6-11) and 35 percent of girls get the recommended amount of regular physical exercise.
- Sadly, only about 8 percent of adolescents (age 12-15) get enough exercise.
- Only 21 percent of adults get enough exercise, according to federal physical activity guidelines for both aerobic and resistance activities.
- 15 percent of adults have great difficulty performing at least one of nine physical activities without help and without the use of special

equipment. The activities that people had trouble performing included: walking a quarter of a mile; climbing 10 steps without resting; standing for 2 hours; sitting for 2 hours; stooping, bending, or kneeling; reaching over their head; using their fingers to grasp small objects; lifting or carrying a 10-pound object; or pushing or pulling large objects.

It would seem that the surge in obesity coupled with a general decline in physical activity has contributed to the dramatic rise in type-II diabetes, which is growing in epidemic proportions. Type-II diabetes, a condition where the body's cells become resistant to insulin, brings on many potential problems, like increased risk of heart disease, stroke, lower limb amputation, and kidney failure. Many obese people, who are not yet diagnosed with type-II diabetes, may already be pre-diabetic, a condition commonly referred to as metabolic syndrome. This condition is characterized by one being obese, having elevated blood-sugar levels, high blood pressure, and high blood triglycerides. What's really sad is that most health experts feel that type-II diabetes and metabolic syndrome could be reversed with proper diet, weight loss, and physical activity – things that we know are good for us. But, even with our current emphasis on diet and exercise, Americans continue to get fatter and physically less fit. We are endangering our health to the point that, for the first time in history, the average life span of the current generation may actually be less than that of the previous generation.

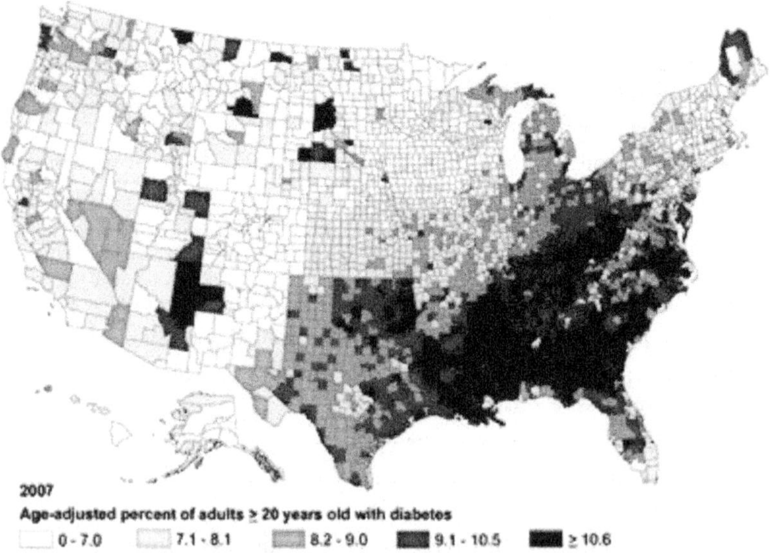

Source: CDC

Our sorry state of fitness could even negatively impact our national security. In recent years our military has had to ease up on the physical conditioning of recruits because so many are now overweight and in bad shape physically. According to a report put out in 2010 by Mission: Readiness (a nonprofit organization), 27 percent of all young adults age 17-24 "are too fat to serve in the military." The report goes on to say that in just a ten-year period from 1998 to 2008, the number of states with 40 percent of young adults being overweight or obese went from only 1 to 39. And in three states – Alabama, Kentucky and Mississippi – over 50 percent of young adults are overweight. Equally alarming is the fact that over 20 percent of recruits failed their initial fitness test.

Clearly, we are missing something. What we are currently doing is not working, since Americans keep getting fatter and less fit. All the diets, gyms, exercise equipment, and fitness gurus have not made one iota of difference in our physical condition. This book lays out a rationale for fitness and a detailed plan for personal physical improvement. To reverse the direction we are headed in, individuals must take control of their lifestyle choices and thus become more responsible for their own physical condition. It won't be easy. You will have to work at it. But, I firmly believe that everyone can improve their physical condition. This book is first and foremost about enhancing your physique. But, I argue that the exercise and dietary habits that help sculpt your physique also lead to all of the recognized benefits attributed to general fitness.

Fitness Philosophy

This book details my personal philosophies of training and nutrition, which can be considered not only a training system but a way of life as well. To build the body you want, you will have to adopt a fitness lifestyle. With my program, you will see results quickly, but you won't be able to maintain those results unless you practice sound habits on a daily basis. This is why most people who lose weight end up gaining it back. Their behaviors didn't change enough to maintain their results. The only approaches that have proved successful in maintaining results involve behavior modifications (lifestyle changes) over the long term. The pursuit of improved fitness delves into three broad areas, with each discussed in much greater detail in the chapters that follow.

- <u>T</u>raining
- <u>N</u>utrition
- <u>T</u>hinking

I refer to these topics as TNT, since, when combined in the correct proportions and utilized properly, they can produce explosive results. Training, the physical aspect of fitness, challenges the body to adapt and become stronger in response to imposed demands. Nutrition involves the food we eat to fuel our body. In addition, it involves how much we eat, when we eat, and the nutrient content of our food. Most people associate fitness with only exercise and nutrition, but the importance of the thinking component cannot be overstated. Everything we do involves thinking, and our thoughts have real power. How we think about our body, for example, determines to a large degree the fitness goals that we decide to pursue. Thinking enables us to evaluate our current condition and then analyze options and make plans for personal improvement. Each of these components is powerful in itself, but combined they create a synergistic program, which is more likely to produce results than when undertaken separately. This powerful, cumulative effect is necessary for one to achieve maximum fitness.

What Exactly Is Exercise?

This question might not be as simple as it first appears. Exercise can be defined as repetitive movement, with a goal in mind, and typically related to improvement in some task or skill or enhancement of physical fitness in general. Even with this definition in mind, all movement can be considered exercise. Washing dishes or your car, gardening, or running the vacuum cleaner, as you probably already know, is exercise. It's work. All movement uses muscles and requires energy. Thus, all movement burns calories above what is required at rest, or what is necessary just to keep you alive. Our bodies were meant to move. Throughout human history, we had to hunt, gather, or grow our food in order to survive, and this took a great deal of movement and work. We just don't move as much today as we used to. Obviously, most of us need to move more, whether that movement is in the form of a coordinated exercise program or simply taking the stairs at work. While all movement can be considered exercise, for the purposes of this book, I am defining exercise as specific activities that are planned with a specific goal in mind and conducted in addition to whatever exercise one engages in on a daily basis through one's job or other regular activities.

In my view, there are no bad forms of exercise, per se. There are, however, certain things some people should not do, based on injuries or physical limitations. If you have heel spurs, for example, you probably should curtail long-distance running. If you have herniated discs in the lumbar region of your back, you shouldn't do barbell squats. So, while all forms of exercise may be beneficial, your exercise program needs to be personalized to suit your particular goals, strengths, and weaknesses.

For the most part, exercise can be divided into two distinct categories:

endurance (often referred to as aerobic or cardio) and resistance (anaerobic). Endurance exercise, like walking, running, and cycling is of low intensity and thus can be done for extended periods of time. This type of training conditions the heart and entire cardiovascular system. And since it can be performed for extended periods of time, endurance training can burn a significant number of calories, which is especially beneficial when trying to lose fat. Resistance exercise, like weightlifting, is higher in intensity and thus is done in short bursts. The primary goal of resistance exercise is to build and maintain muscle mass. The two forms of exercise often overlap. If you increase the intensity of aerobic movements, for example, as in the case of running becoming sprinting, then it can only be done in short bursts and begins to offer some of the same results as resistance exercise. On the other hand, if you decrease the intensity of resistance exercise, it can become more aerobic in nature, as in the case of using light weight and performing higher reps or doing several exercises in a row, commonly referred to as circuit training.

A Brief History of Exercise and Fitness

Exercise, as I am defining here, is a relatively recent activity for humans. For most of human history, life has required hard physical work, consisting mainly of hunting and gathering food. It would have been unthinkable for someone of the middle ages or even as recent as the early 20th century to go for a jog with the intent of enhancing one's fitness. People played – as in swimming or games – but these kinds of activities were seen as leisure and not so much as exercise. In other words, people didn't do them to burn off excess calories or condition their cardiovascular system. Today, people actually pay money to exercise. Of course, many people pay a hefty gym fee and still don't exercise.

The ancient Greeks believed in the proper balance between mind and body and gave us images of the ideal physique. Persia, Sparta, and Rome advocated the importance of physical fitness but primarily as a means to prepare young men to be stronger, more fit, warriors. In fact, throughout history war and military preparation has spurred periods of increased emphases on fitness among nations. Modern gymnastics came into prominence in Europe in the 1700s, which led to the establishment of exercise facilities and an increased emphasis on fitness for the general population. America's participation in two world wars brought the importance of fitness into the public's consciousness. I place the emergence of the fitness culture early in the 20th century, when people began to make the connection between exercise and nutrition and overall health. Jack LeLanne was America's first true fitness guru. In the early 50s he was the first to utilize television to bring fitness programming to the masses. The early 70s saw several important developments come together that helped to launch the modern fitness movement. The whole aerobics craze we see today only came into existence in the early 1970s, based on the work of Dr. Kenneth Cooper. Barbells and dumbbells came into existence in the 1930s, but the 70s saw exercise machines begin to dot the fitness landscape. Arthur Jones invented Nautilus and built an empire by promoting his machines and his philosophy of brief but high-intensity exercise. Perhaps the most influential individual in the fitness movement was Joe Weider. Joe popularized bodybuilding through his magazines, and one of his early stars, Arnold Schwarzenegger, put bodybuilding on the map in the mid-70s and later muscled in on movie fame. Sports teams didn't realize and take advantage of the benefits of weightlifting until at least the 70s. Up until then coaches and trainers actually thought that weightlifting would hinder athletic performance by making players muscle bound, a term denoting inflexibility, reduced speed and diminished agility. Since the beginning of the modern fitness movement, circa 1970, popular fitness has been dominated by one fad after another.

The Benefits of Exercise

We've known for a long time that exercise, of any type, is good for us. Our bodies were meant to move – to work. We have legs and feet designed for walking and running long distances. We have upper bodies designed for pulling, pushing, lifting, and carrying objects. We have also known for some time now that regular exercise enhances health, increases longevity, and contributes to a higher quality of life. Exercise may be the closest thing to the elusive fountain of youth. In fact, exercise has been shown to be somewhat of a cure-all, contributing to longevity, while enhancing mood, energy, and sleep. And there's nothing that elevates our self-esteem and self-confidence more than having an aesthetically-pleasing physique.

It's really true that a sound body makes for a sound mind. It's little surprise, then, that more people than ever are interested in improving their body, fitness level, and overall health. Most New Year's resolutions, for example, involve weight-loss and/or more exercise. In fact, it's hard to imagine any self-improvement program not involving the pursuit of fitness. Obviously, it's challenging, since so many never reach their fitness goals. If it were easy, everyone would have a great physique and a high level of fitness. It's hard work, but the potential payoff can be life-fulfilling, as well as life-extending. Those who exercise regularly can look forward to many of the following rewards:

- A lower body weight.
- A stronger immune system, which means your body is better able

to fight off illnesses. A stronger immune system also means that you can recover more quickly from illnesses and injuries.

- Reduced risk of cancer, heart disease, diabetes, and other major diseases.
- Improved cardiovascular health.
- A more efficient metabolism.
- Higher levels of good cholesterol, and lower levels of bad cholesterol.
- Improved mental health, including decreased depression, stress, and anxiety.
- Improved cognitive ability, which includes less risk of developing Alzheimer's later in life.
- Better, more restful sleep.
- A longer, more productive lifespan.

Which Type of Exercise is Best?

Let me state right up front possibly the most important principle of my philosophy of fitness – one that you will hear many times throughout this book: **Any exercise is better than no exercise**. In almost all cases, doing something is better than doing nothing. This is the type of thinking that spawned the famous Nike slogan "Just do it." However, simply saying that all exercise is good is not all that helpful for people wanting to improve their level of fitness. Just do what? In order to reach and maintain high levels of fitness, people need reliable information about how to structure an effective fitness program. One must include, for example, both endurance and resistance exercise, but how much of each?

It's often difficult to categorize exercises as being purely aerobic or resistance. There are many exercises that fall between these two ends of the spectrum. Walking is closer to the aerobic end while sprinting is closer to the anaerobic end. Weight training with very high reps is more aerobic in nature. So, the whole question of aerobic versus resistance doesn't tell the whole story. For me, it's more a question of balance and priorities. If you only had time for one type of exercise, then I would favor resistance training. You can get the benefits of aerobic exercise through resistance training, but the reverse in not true. You can't build muscle by doing only endurance-type exercise. Therefore, I advocate a program centered around resistance training and supplemented with endurance-type training. I refer to this system of training as the cerebral approach, with "cerebral" associated with an emphasis on critical thinking.

What's the Best Training Method to Get into Shape?

A vigorous five-mile walk will do more good for an unhappy but otherwise healthy adult than all the medicine and psychology in the world. – Paul Dudley White

Although not directly stated, the question also implies efficiency in addition to productivity. Which training methods will get you where you want to be in the shortest amount of time? The answer depends somewhat on your goals. Some people, for instance, might simply want to do some regular cardio training to improve their heart health and may not be looking for a total body transformation. For many people, walking is the perfect exercise, since it's relatively easy and inexpensive to do. Honestly, any exercise done on a regular basis can be part of an effective fitness plan. However, many people desire to lose bodyfat and gain muscle – in other words – to change how their body looks. Some use the word "toned" when referring to their muscles, but what they are really referring to is building their muscles and stripping away bodyfat so the muscles become more visible. Which specific group of people has this type of look? Right, bodybuilders. So, to achieve a more muscular and leaner look, most people should train more like bodybuilders. They should lift weights three or four days a week and do cardio sessions also about three or four days a week.

I understand that the bodybuilder look is not desired by everyone. Well, don't worry. It's very unlikely that you will end up as big and lean as a bodybuilder simply because you emulate their training. Most competitive bodybuilders – the ones you see on the covers of muscle magazines – have superior genetics for building muscle and staying lean. What you can do, though, is to gain an appreciable amount of muscle while losing a significant amount of fat, which, as a result, will dramatically enhance your physique.

For someone wanting to dramatically change how they look, by adding muscle and losing fat, I recommend training daily but not doing the same workout every day. I advocate daily training as a means to develop good habits and to keep your metabolism at a high level. You should engage in some sort of exercise each and every day. Keep in mind that "training" could consist of heavy weightlifting or light cardio, like walking a mile or two. In fact, it's counterproductive to train hard every day. You shouldn't train with weights every day, for example. If you lift hard and heavy, as you should, it's just too much stress on the body to do every day, even if you don't work the same muscle groups every time you train. Some people overdo cardio work, too. Take a good look at people who train for marathons and triathlons, for example. They are lean, even gaunt, and have very little muscle. Too much endurance training interferes with muscle development. These people don't look very healthy to me, and I believe it is due to their being so grossly over-trained.

I recommend joining a gym and here's why: 1) Most gyms have a wide variety of equipment, which will bring more variety to your workouts. 2) Training with others who have common goals can be a strong motivator. 3) A gym is a good place to learn more about training. You can work with a trainer or simply watch and talk to others. Just be wary of those who always seem to offer unsolicited advice; many of these individuals don't know what they're doing. People can meet their fitness goals by training at home, but I think it is more challenging. First off, most home exercise equipment goes unused, unless you count it as a clothes hanger. And so much of the equipment marketed for home use is of low quality or outright junk. It's just too hard to stay motivated at home. There's often not enough space, not enough equipment, and too many distractions, like the couch or recliner. The gym is a much better atmosphere for training, and, everything accounted for, not that expensive. For about a dollar a day you can have access to a myriad of high-quality weight and cardio machines, free weights, and perhaps classes. If you are serious about maximizing fitness and reshaping your body, you need to be hitting the gym on a regular basis.

How Much Exercise?

The answer to this question depends on at least a couple of important factors: 1) The type of exercise and 2) The intensity of the exercise. Generally, more exercise is better than less, but only up to a point. This is where the intensity of the exercise becomes a crucial consideration. The higher the intensity of exercise, the greater the demands (stress) placed on the body. Therefore, to avoid overtraining, high intensity exercise – like heavy resistance work – must be brief and relatively infrequent. Low-intensity exercise – like walking or housework – can be carried on much longer without any threat of overtraining. Low-intensity exercise is more likely to lead to monotony, and that's why people can stand only so much of it.

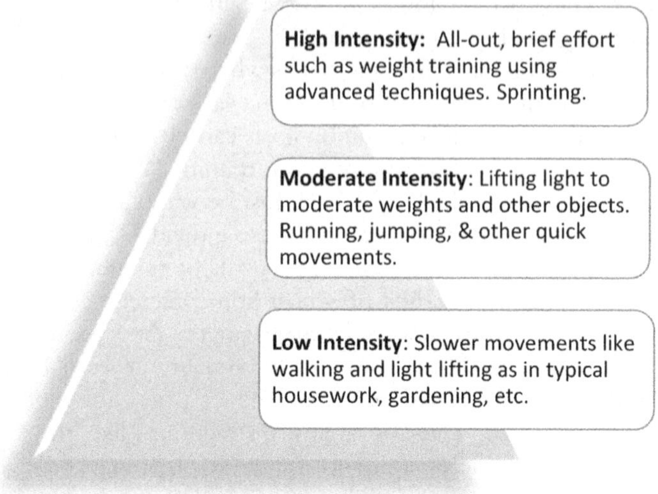

Distribution of Intensity on a Daily and Weekly Basis			
Time Frame	**Low**	**Moderate**	**High**
Daily (in hours)	5-6 hours	1-2 hours	1/2 hour
Weekly (in days)	Daily	6 days	4 days
Total Hours/Week	35 hours	12 hours	2 hours

Since almost all daily activities involve relatively slow and easy movement, most of your exercise will fall into the low-intensity category. Most people can tolerate several hours of low-intensity exercise on a daily basis, but this level of exercise tends to become monotonous or boring. Being somewhat more demanding, moderate-level exercise can't, and shouldn't, be done for as long as low-intensity exercise. Most peoples' workouts fall into this category, since most people can build up to this intensity but will not force themselves into the high-intensity zone. Only brief bouts of high-intensity exercise can be tolerated without overtraining. This type of exercise shouldn't be done more than 4 days per week, and then no more than 30 minutes at a time. You might think that since your high-intensity workouts last an hour that you are overtraining. Probably not. Keep in mind that after you do a high-intense set, you typically rest for a minute or so. So, during a normal workout, rest time equals or likely exceeds actual work time.

It's important to remember that all exercise is cumulative and thus must be managed. Obviously, high-intensity exercise must be kept to a minimum, due to the severe demands it places on the body. Working backwards, the bulk of your moderate exercise should be conducted on the days when you do no high-intensity exercise at all. Since we get most of our low-intensity exercise at our jobs, this variable might be out of our control. However, many people now have jobs that require very little exercise. In these cases, people need to find ways to increase their time doing low-intensity exercise.

The Cerebral Approach: Bodybuilding With a Twist

Bodybuilders are extreme athletes. I'm not saying that you need to train and eat exactly like hard-core bodybuilders. That is both unrealistic and unnecessary. I simply want you to emulate some of the things that bodybuilders do, since bodybuilders are the best examples we have of how to build muscle. And building muscle should be your main concern. The fitness-enhancing program that I advocate is what I refer to as the cerebral approach, due to the fact that I place such a high priority on critical thinking. In essence, my cerebral approach takes the best aspects of bodybuilding and leaves out those practices that are not supported by science or that may be dangerous or otherwise nonproductive. My cerebral approach includes short bursts of intense resistance exercise, for example, because that is what has been shown in numerous studies to produce the greatest results in muscle hypertrophy. The cerebral approach, however, does not advocate ingesting massive amounts of protein, which is a common practice among bodybuilders, but not supported by nutrition science and may even be dangerous.

Fitness can be achieved through a variety of means, but the most effective and efficient approach is to combine various training methods into a comprehensive program. Being a bodybuilder myself, my training approach emphasizes intense weight training, as this is a must for building muscle. Building muscle is the only way to change the way your body looks. Losing fat only makes you smaller. Your body still looks the same, and sometimes people who lose weight, without doing any resistance work, actually end up looking worse than they did before. People talk about being "toned," as if this is some special condition that muscles take on due to training. What toned actually means is that muscles have become slightly bigger while also losing some bodyfat around them so they become more noticeable. By having more muscle you will burn more calories, even at rest. We tend to lose muscle and bone mass as we age, a process that many researchers believe contributes greatly to the frailties of old age. In fact, many researchers think that this gradual loss of muscle is a primary contributor to the aging process. The good news is that regular resistance exercise significantly slows this process and thus has the potential to enhance the quality of life of not only seniors but everyone as well. The tangible benefits of resistance exercise are many:

- Increased bone mass
- Increased strength
- Muscle gain
- Fat loss
- Higher metabolism
- Enhanced self-esteem
- Stress reduction
- Increased longevity
- Improvement in sports performance

In addition to intense weight training, the cerebral approach includes a healthy dose of cardio exercise, since it is the most efficient means for conditioning the cardiovascular system. The cerebral approach is also a holistic approach, which entails exercise, diet, critical thinking, and attitudes. The cerebral approach is very close to the common term "wellness," which incorporates the physical, mental, and even spiritual components of life. Maybe the best way to describe the cerebral approach is to call it a fitness lifestyle, or fitness as a philosophy of life. In this way, we consciously choose behaviors that contribute to enhanced fitness. Then, over time, these behaviors become engrained habits that are second nature to us. And like all self-improvement, the fitness lifestyle encourages us to continually strive toward improving our fitness.

Why People Are So Averse to Exercise: The Law of Conservation of Energy

People cite all kinds of excuses for not exercising as much as they should, with the most common one being lack of time. While this is true for some, it doesn't fully answer the question as to why so many don't like to exercise and, like other forms of work, avoid it like the plague. I have a theory as to why this behavior is so prevalent among most people (and, really, all animals) and always has been. Borrowing a scientific term, I call it the conservation of energy. In physics, the law of conservation of energy states that energy can neither be created nor destroyed. Energy can be converted from one form to another, but the amount of energy in a closed system remains constant. The food we eat contains energy that is either converted into glucose for immediate energy or stored as fat for use when incoming energy (food) is low. The amount of fat we have depends upon the balance of energy coming in, in the form of food, versus the amount of energy we use, in the form of work, exercise, metabolism, and other bodily functions like breathing, which keeps us alive. Throughout this complicated process, though, the amount of energy doesn't change.

Humans, like other animals, conserve energy primarily due to the fact that our lives depend upon this precarious balance between calories in versus calories used. I contend that our bodies have been programmed, via evolution, to not waste energy. From the beginning of human history we have had to expend energy gathering energy, i.e. food to eat and fuel to keep us warm. There were times when food and fuel were scarce, and therefore our energy stores dwindled to dangerously low levels. In essence, the success of the human species has been about pursuing, using, and conserving energy. Due to periodic famines and the inconsistency of food sources, our bodies became very efficient at storing energy – fat. From that standpoint, it would have been unwise to waste that stored energy on activities that did not result in the acquisition of more energy. And that's why people today avoid all excess movement. Over the millennia, these behaviors became embedded deeply in our genetic makeup. Now still lurking in our unconscious, our brains tell us that exercise is a waste of valuable energy. It also explains why most people, in general, are somewhat lazy, due again to conservation of energy. We see the same behaviors throughout the animal kingdom. Predators expend most of their energy stalking and running down their prey. When they are not hunting, they are laying around. Just observe your cat or dog for a while, and you'll see what I mean. You've no doubt heard how busy bees are. As it turns out, bees are idle about 70 percent of the time. It appears as though energy conservation within the animal kingdom is a natural phenomenon, one that impacts humans as much as any other species.

A second major consideration of the law of conservation of energy involves the body's preference to maintain homeostasis, which centers around a balance of energy out versus energy in. In other words, the body attempts to maintain a constant weight. That's why your metabolism decreases in response to a drastic drop in caloric intake. Your body senses this drop in incoming energy and adjusts itself to utilize less energy. Similarly, if you use more energy by doing more exercise, your body senses this, too, and responds by increasing your appetite so you will eat more and thus make up the energy deficit. You may also be inclined to rest more and move less in response to an increase in exercise, which, again, serves to conserve energy and maintain homeostasis.

And finally, there is a somewhat mysterious fact regarding the health benefits of exercise that rarely gets any attention and few people even know about. It appears as though regular exercise is not healthy for all individuals. A recent study looking at common health measures of those engaged in regular exercise found that a full 10 percent of test subjects experienced adverse changes in one or more of the following heart disease markers: resting systolic blood pressure, HDL cholesterol, triglycerides, and insulin.

Why Do Some People Like to Exercise?

While I have just argued why most people avoid exercise, there are those few who actually like to exercise. I say few. There are lots of people who like to exercise, but they are certainly in the minority. Exercise has been shown to affect brain chemicals, like dopamine, for example. Dopamine is a feel-good chemical, so this explains why many experience euphoric-like feelings while exercising. It also explains why some actually get addicted to exercise. I experience these high feelings when I work out. I love the feeling I get when I feel my muscles working. Arnold Schwarzenegger once compared the feeling of the pump to an orgasm. I don't know if I would go quite that far, but I know where he is coming from. The question is why don't more people experience the types of good feelings that I do while training?

It's also true that we tend to do what we are good at. Some people are simply good at working out. It seems to come naturally for them. They are able to make good progress, while others, less gifted, struggle. Some feel good while training; others feel nothing but pain, during and after training. I admit that I love being in the gym. It is an environment that I excel in. I get a lot of respect and deference there. I get many compliments on my physique and questions from those who are trying to build theirs. All this positive attention only adds to the good feelings I get while training at the gym. We all seek out environments that reward us, but for many, the gym offers few rewards, and thus people feel out of place and uncomfortable.

The Role of Genetics

Each component of fitness is attainable, at least to some degree, for all of us, but we have to work at them . . . some of us more so than others. This book is all about what you can do to realize your physical potential, and believe me, you can and should do a lot in that regard. However, you already know that people are different, with vastly different physical characteristics and potentials. As much as I want you to work hard, develop good habits, and think positively, I'd be lying to you if I told you that your results will be totally under your direct control. Like other personal traits, our genes play an important role in determining our health and overall fitness. We know that all sorts of diseases and conditions, for example, run in families, making it much more likely that it will impact certain individuals sometime in their lifetime. Genes play a role in longevity, for example. Some people seem to be destined to live much longer than average, even when they don't take particularly good care of themselves. And genes determine to a great extent our fitness potential. No matter how hard we work, few of us are ever going to be professional athletes. As with other talents, some people are simply gifted. Few of us are ever going to have six-pack abs, or be competitive in a bodybuilding competition or a marathon. However, that doesn't mean we shouldn't try. If anything, it means that we should try harder. We all have much more potential than we realize, and we should push the limits to see what we can do. One thing is certain: we can all improve our overall fitness, if we work at it. We can become stronger, leaner, increase our endurance, and, ultimately, be healthier and happier. I challenge you to try.

Perspective

Exercise is the key to fitness, and any exercise is better than no exercise. Anyone can make progress, regardless of their genetic makeup, but how do we get more people to exercise? Why do some people like to exercise while others can't stand it? I'm not saying that everyone has to like to exercise. That's not realistic. Maybe the best we can do is to make exercise a higher priority, but how? We haven't looked at the deterioration of fitness as a threat to our species, but I firmly believe it is that serious.

2. ASSESSING FITNESS

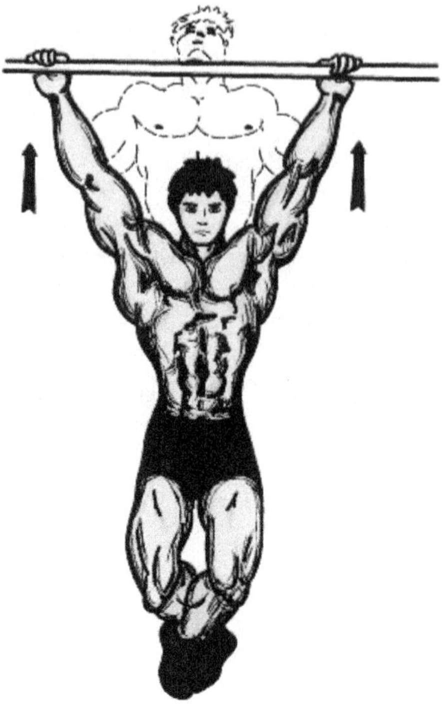

Physical fitness is not only one of the most important keys to a healthy body, it is the basis of dynamic and creative intellectual ability.
– John F. Kennedy

On May 6, 1954, Englishman Roger Bannister did something rather remarkable, something that no one, as far as we know, had ever accomplished up to that point in history. On that spring day, Bannister, a 25-year-old medical student at Oxford, became the first human to run a mile in less than 4 minutes. Up to that point, many thought that a sub-4-minute mile was physically impossible – that the human body was simply incapable of doing it. To put the feat into perspective, to break the 4-

minute barrier, one has to run slightly faster than 15 miles per hour for nearly 4 minutes. Needless to say, it is a nearly unfathomable feat of physical fitness . . . and of will.

Ironically, only a few weeks after Bannister broke the 4-minute barrier, another runner broke his record, and within just 3 years, 16 runners had also broken the once seemingly impossible barrier. The current record in the mile is a whole 15 seconds faster than Bannister's. It seems as though every few years someone shaves another second off the time, setting a new record. This makes me wonder just what is humanly possible. Is a 3-minute mile possible? Records are broken each year in all sorts of physical feats. Just recently, someone bench pressed 1,000 lbs., which was once thought unattainable. My point is that we continue to push our physical limits as a species. We (some of us) get faster, stronger, and more agile. It's ironic that as a few near superhumans continue to break records, overall fitness of the general populations continues to decline. Most individuals will never set world records, but we can certainly improve our physical prowess and attain higher levels of fitness.

We all want to be healthy and vibrant. We want to be strong and lean, to look good and feel good. I'll admit that I'd like to be superhuman, like Bannister. Who wants to be average? I want to stand out in the crowd. But what is average? This chapter identifies specific objective measures of fitness, how they can be assessed, and what levels are considered average. Objective measures of fitness allow us to test ourselves, compare ourselves to others, and also serve to motivate us. We see what is possible in others and think about our own potential.

What does it mean to be fit? Here's a short list of measures that are typically indicative of one's level of fitness:

- Body-fat percentage
- Body weight
- Body-Mass Index (BMI): There's an optimal range from 22-26.
- Resting pulse rate: Lower is considered healthier.
- Time it takes you to run/walk a mile
- Number of pushups performed in one minute
- Number of situps performed in one minute
- Number of pullups performed in one minute
- Amount of weight lifted for one rep in the bench press
- Number of repetitions performed in the bench press using one's own body weight

Let's look at these measures in more detail. What's average and what's super fit?

1. **Bodyfat percentage**: The amount of fat on/in your body versus your lean mass, with lower levels indicating greater fitness. Average levels for men range from 15 to 20 percent and 20 to 25 percent for women. Competitive bodybuilders get as low as 3 percent, an insanely low level that can be maintained for only very short periods of time. Elite athletes typically fall in the range of 6 to 12 percent.
2. **Bodyweight**: How much you weigh. Weight correlates highly with body-fat percentage, except in cases of individuals with a high level of muscle mass, like bodybuilders and other elite athletes. Weight should be monitored closely, but with the premise that one's body-fat percentage tells much more about overall body composition and fitness.
3. **Body-Mass Index (BMI)**: The BMI is a number that takes into account your weight and your height. Like weight alone, though, it still doesn't account for varying levels of muscle mass, which skews one's weight. The range for optimal fitness is between 21 and 24.

	Normal Range				Overweight Range					Obese Range			
BMI	21	22	23	24	25	26	27	28	29	30	31	32	33
Height (inches)	Weight (pounds)												
4'10"	100	105	110	115	119	124	129	134	138	143	148	153	158
4'11"	104	109	114	119	124	128	133	138	143	148	153	158	163
5'0"	107	112	118	123	128	133	138	143	148	153	158	163	168
5'1"	111	116	122	127	132	137	143	148	153	158	164	169	174
5'2"	115	120	126	131	136	142	147	153	158	164	169	175	180
5'3"	118	124	130	135	141	146	152	158	163	169	175	180	186
5'4"	122	128	134	140	145	151	157	163	169	174	180	186	192
5'5"	126	132	138	144	150	156	162	168	174	180	186	192	198
5'6"	130	136	142	148	155	161	167	173	179	186	192	198	204
5'7"	134	140	146	153	159	166	172	178	185	191	198	204	211
5'8"	138	144	151	158	164	171	177	184	190	197	203	210	216
5'9"	142	149	155	162	169	176	182	189	196	203	209	216	223
5'10"	146	153	160	167	174	181	188	195	202	209	216	222	229
5'11"	150	157	165	172	179	186	193	200	208	215	222	229	236
6'0"	150	157	165	172	179	186	193	200	208	215	222	235	242
6'1"	159	166	174	182	189	197	204	212	219	227	235	242	250
6'2"	163	171	179	186	194	202	210	218	225	233	241	249	256
6'3"	168	176	184	192	200	208	216	224	232	240	248	256	264

(Weight is measured with underclothes and no shoes.)

4. **Resting pulse rate (RPR)**: The heart of the average person beats

about 70 to 75 times per minute at rest and of course much faster at times, in response to one's physical activity. The heart must pump oxygen-rich blood to all parts of the body. The heart of a more fit person can do this job more efficiently and thus requires fewer beats to do the same amount of work. Elite endurance athletes have RPRs in the low to mid 40s. Now that is superhuman.

5. **Time to run/walk 1 mile**: This event measures one's endurance and thus indicates how efficient your cardiovascular system is at delivering oxygen to all parts of the body. If you run/walk a mile in less than 8 minutes, you're in pretty good shape. If you can do it in less than 6 minutes, you're in tremendous shape. 4 minutes or under and you're superhuman.
6. **Number of pushups performed in 1 minute**: This event measures your upper-body pushing strength and endurance. 40 in 1 minute is good; 50 is great; and 60 or more is outstanding.
7. **Number of situps performed in 1 minute**: Measures the strength and endurance of your abdominal muscles. 60 in a minute is good; 80 is great; 100 or more is outstanding.
8. **Number of pullups performed in 1 minute**: Measures your upper-body pulling strength and endurance. 10 is good; 15 is great; 18 or more is in the superhuman range.
9. **Number of dips performed in 1 minute**: Measures all-around upper-body strength and endurance. 15 is good; 25 is great; 30 or more is outstanding. For a description of the dip, see Chapter 13.
10. **1-rep maximum on the bench press**: Measures pure upper-body strength/power. Benching your bodyweight is considered good; 1.5 x your bodyweight is great; and doubling your bodyweight gets you into the superhuman category.
11. **Total repetitions performed in the bench press using one's bodyweight**: Perhaps the best measure of pure upper-body strength and endurance. Approximately 50 percent of men can't even bench their own bodyweight once. This is the primary method the NFL combine uses to test the strength of potential draft choices. Benching your bodyweight for more than one rep is good; 10 reps is great; and 20 or more is approaching superhuman.
12. **1-rep maximum in the deadlift:** Arguably, the deadlift is the best measure of overall strength and power, since the exercise involves so many muscles. The deadlift is so effective at building muscle, strength, and power that it is used by powerlifters, bodybuilders, crossfitters, and other athletes as well. Deadlifting 1.5 x your bodyweight is good; 2 x your bodyweight is excellent; and 3 x your bodyweight is superhuman.
13. **Total repetitions performed in the Deadlift using one's body-**

weight: Because the deadlift is so demanding, performing several repetitions really taxes both your muscular and cardiovascular systems. Doing more than 10 reps becomes a pretty effective cardio workout. Being able to get 10 reps with your bodyweight is good; 20 reps is great; and more than 25 reps puts you in the league of superhumans.

When I was in the Army, my physical training test consisted of timed push-ups, sit-ups, and a two-mile run. The Marines have a similar test, with pull-ups included.

A Note on Gender Differences

We can't simply ignore the fact that gender differences exist. Men, on the whole, are simply bigger, stronger, and faster than women. This doesn't mean, though, that women should train any differently than men. It does, however, make it difficult to compare men and women's performances on certain exercises. The specific exercises I'm referring to from above are pushups, and pullups. Lacking upper body strength, women struggle pushing or pulling their bodyweight. Women can make exceptional progress in building strength, but in the beginning, it's going to be difficult. None of the women at my gym, for instance, not even the fittest ones, can do a single unassisted pullup. Because of this strength liability, I recommend women do girl pushups – the ones where the knees are on the floor – until enough upper-body strength is built to allow for regular pushups. Similarly, I recommend that women start out doing assisted pullups. These can be done by having a spotter provide just enough assistance to get you up far enough. Many gyms have a machine that does this for you.

How Healthy Are You?

Health is more than how you feel or look, even though these things tell us much about our degree of health. Obviously, health and fitness overlap quite a bit, meaning that health is a major part of fitness, and fitness is a major part of health. The two even share many measures. One of the primary goals of any fitness program, for example, should be to enhance overall health. And there's ample evidence that the best way to enhance overall health is to engage in regular exercise, consume a healthy diet, and think positively.

For the most part, optimal health describes a condition whereby the body's systems are 1) free of disease; and 2) performing at a high level. What sort of measures can help us assess our overall health? Below is a short list of common health indicators, with their optimal levels. Being outside the normal ranges may be indicative of disease or malfunction.

1. **Blood Pressure**: It is estimated that approximately 40 percent of the adult U.S. population currently has high blood pressure, which is a reading exceeding 140/90. Another 30 percent have borderline or prehypertension, which is a reading that exceeds 130/80. An ideal reading is 120/70. Blood pressure has been called the "silent killer," since people with it might never have any symptoms until it has done considerable damage to their health. High blood pressure is a major contributing factor in heart and kidney disease and stroke.

Blood Pressure Classification	Systolic Blood Pressure (top number)	Diastolic Blood Pressure (bottom number)
Normal	<120	and <80
Prehypertension	120-139	or 80-89
Stage I Hypertension	140-159	or 90-99
Stage II Hypertension	>160	or >100

2. **BMI**: As discussed above, BMI has its flaws but is relatively predictive of overall health for the majority of the population.
3. **Waist:** One's waist measurement is somewhat predictive of future disease, with higher measurements being linked to heart disease and diabetes. Visceral (abdominal) fat is related to insulin resistance, metabolic syndrome, diabetes, and cardiovascular disease. A waist measurement over 40 inches for men, and 35 inches for women, puts one at a much greater risk of disease.
4. **Waist to Hip Ratio**: This measure is somewhat predictive of disease, since where a person stores fat – the hips or waist – says a lot about one's relative risk of disease. Generally, a higher waist to hip ratio puts one at greater risk of diabetes and cardiovascular disease. Ratios greater than 0.8 for women and 1.0 for men are associated with an increased risk of disease.
5. **Resting Heart Rate (RHR)**: As stated above, the RHR tells a lot about what's going on with one's cardiovascular system. A lower RHR is indicative of a more efficient cardiovascular system.

Other measures are worth monitoring as well by analyzing one's blood and/or urine. It should be noted that the results of these measures can vary with age, level and type of activity, medications you are currently taking, etc. Make sure to discuss the results with your doctor.

Common Indicators/Markers of Health		
Measure	**Description**	**Normal Range**
Glucose	A measure of the amount of sugar in the blood, which indicates how well insulin is functioning in the body to remove sugar from the blood. High levels may be indicative of pre-diabetes or diabetes.	70 – 110 mg/dl
Bilirubin	A yellowish pigment found in bile, a fluid produced by the liver. Bilirubin is a by-product from the breakdown of heme as older red blood cells are replaced by new ones. The liver helps break down bilirubin so it can be excreted via the stool. High levels can cause jaundice and is indicative of several diseases, including those affecting the liver.	0.2 – 1.9 mg/dl
Creatinine	A waste product formed from the breakdown of creatine, which is central to the production of energy for working muscles. Creatinine in the blood is filtered by the kidneys and excreted through urine. High levels in the blood may be indicative of impaired kidney function.	0.8 – 1.4 mg/dl
Liver Enzymes	The following enzymes are typically associated with liver function.	
ALT	Alanine Aminotransferase is an enzyme contained in cells of the liver. High levels may signal a diseased or distressed liver.	5 – 65 U/L
AST	Aspartate Aminotransferase is an enzyme in all cells of the body. It is elevated typically as a result of liver or muscle damage.	0 – 37 U/L

Electrolytes	This test shows the levels of specific electrolytes, such as sodium, potassium, and chloride, and whether an imbalance exists among them. Such an imbalance can have adverse effects on several body systems, such as blood pressure, kidney function, and heart rate.	
Sodium	An essential mineral contained in every cell of the body. High levels are associated with dehydration, heart disease, excessive intake of dietary salt, or diabetes insipidus.	136 – 145 mmol/L
Potassium	An essential mineral regulated by the kidneys. It helps with the communication between muscles and nerves and helps to move nutrients into cells. High levels are associated with dehydration.	3.5 – 5.1 mmol/L
Chloride	Works with the other electrolytes to keep the body's ph level and fluids balanced. Chloride levels usually correspond to sodium levels.	98 – 107 mmol/L
Carbon Dioxide (Co2)	A by-product of cellular metabolism and an indirect measure of bicarbonate in the blood, which is indicative of the blood's buffering capacity. Higher levels could be the result of acid production in the blood.	21 – 32 mmol/L
BUN	Blood urea nitrogen. Nitrogen is excreted by the kidneys as a result of the breakdown of protein. The test is used to test kidney function, as high BUN levels may be indicative of excessive stress on the kidneys.	7 – 20 mg/dl
BUN/ Creatinine Ratio	High ratios suggest dehydration, possible kidney malfunction, or high protein consumption. Low ratios suggest kidney or liver diseases, malnutrition, or Sickle Cell Anemia.	10:1 – 20:1
Total Protein	The total protein test measures the total amount of two classes of	6.3 – 7.9 g/dl

	proteins found in the fluid portion of your blood.	
Albumin	Albumin is the most abundant protein contained in human plasma. It transports hormones, lipids, and other compounds, helps to buffer ph and maintain osmotic pressure. Low albumin levels may be indicative of liver or kidney problems.	3.9 – 5.0 g/dl
Lipid Profile	Lipids are types of fats in the blood. Includes total cholesterol, HDL, LDL, and triglycerides (fat in the blood).	
Total Cholesterol	Cholesterol is a fatty substance produced mainly by the liver and ingested in the animal products we eat, like meat and eggs. Cholesterol is vital to the body as it is contained in each cell membrane and is used by the body to produce bile acids and steroid hormones such as testosterone, estradiol, progesterone, and cortisol. Excess cholesterol can build up in the walls of arteries, which can eventually lead to hardening of the arteries and restricted blood flow. A heart attack usually occurs when a cholesterol plaque ruptures within a coronary artery causing a blood clot to form which cuts off the flow of blood to a particular part of the heart. High cholesterol is associated with an increased risk of heart disease.	Less than 200 mg/dl: desirable; 200 – 239: borderline
HDL	High-density lipoprotein (good cholesterol). Circulating in the bloodstream, its larger size actually helps to keep plaques from forming in arteries that could impede or cut off blood flow to the heart or brain. Therefore, the higher number the better off you are.	Women: >50 Men: >40
LDL	Low-density lipoprotein (bad cholesterol). The smaller size of these	<129: good 130 – 159:

	particles contributes to their buildup on artery walls, and thus creating dangerous plaques that can choke off blood flow or break off and completely obstruct the flow of blood. Therefore, high levels of LDL cholesterol are associated with an increased risk of heart disease and stroke.	borderline >159: high
VLDL	Very low-density lipoprotein (very bad cholesterol). Due to their very small size, these particles are likely to wreak havoc in our arteries. Obviously, the lower the number the better.	<30
Triglycerides	These are fat particles (lipids) in the blood. Excess calories (from all food we eat) are converted into triglycerides and stored in our fat cells. High levels of triglycerides is associated with obesity, metabolic syndrome, and diabetes. High levels are a risk factor for heart disease and stroke.	<150: desirable 150 – 199: borderline >199: high
Hormone Levels	Hormones regulate all sorts of bodily functions. So when a particular hormone is out of whack, it usually causes some sort of malfunction in one or more systems of the body. Therefore, hormone levels can tell us a lot about what's going on in our body.	Men (Testosterone) Women (Estrogen) (progesterone)
Inflammation in the Body	Typically measured by the amount of C-reactive protein (CRP) found in the blood. A high degree of inflammation in the body can do significant damage to several major bodily systems, and thus is thought to be a primary cause of many diseases.	0 – 1.0 mg/L

The Fitness Index

For those who really want to challenge themselves and compare their level of fitness to others, I came up with what I call the Fitness Index. The Fitness Index scores your performance on several of the measures listed previously in this chapter allowing you to arrive at a grand total, or index, which can then be compared to others' scores. See the table below to see how to derive your index score.

Fitness Index

Measure	Description	Points	Score
Pushups	The number of pushups completed in 1 minute	1 point for each rep completed	
Situps	The number of situps completed in 1 minute	1 point for each rep completed	
Dips	The number of dips completed in 1 minute	1 point for each rep completed	
Pullups	The number of pullups completed in 1 minute	1 point for each rep completed	
Bench Press x Bodyweight	The number of reps completed in 1 minute using one's bodyweight	2 points for each rep completed	
Deadlift x Bodyweight	The number of reps completed in 1 minute using one's bodyweight	2 points for each rep completed	
Subtotal	Scores of above measures added together		
1-Mile Run/Walk	The time it takes to run/walk 1 mile	Total time x 2 and that number subtracted from the subtotal	
Grand Total	Subtotal minus score for 1-mile run/walk		

Rating Scale

<41 = Below Average
41 – 70 = Average
71 – 100 = Good
101 – 140 = Excellent
141 – 180 = Remarkable
181 – 220 = Freakish
221 and above = Superhuman

Here's an example of how to derive your score: Let's say a trainee performed 30 pushups, 40 situps, 10 dips, 4 pullups, 5 reps on bench, 6 reps on deadlift, and did the 1-mile run in 8:30. His/her score would be 30+40+10+4+10+12-17=89. This puts him/her in the "good" category, as this is a respectable score.

The seven exercises must be done as one event, separated by no more than a five-minute rest period. The order of the exercises can be altered, but the run must do done last. All scores must be witnessed and verified by at least one other person. It may be best to do the exercises as a group event.

Modifications for Women

Obviously, the Fitness Index is kinder to men than to women, due mainly to the advantage men have in upper-body strength. I certainly don't want to leave women out of this, so here are the modifications I recommend for women to score themselves on each exercise:

Pushup: Perform girl pushups.
Situp: No modification necessary. Women should be able to perform almost equally with men on this one.
Dip: Do assisted dips on the machine made for this at the gym. And set the pin on the machine so that you are pushing about three-quarters of your bodyweight. If you don't have access to this machine, Use your legs to boost yourself up and then lower yourself under your own power.
Pullup: Basically the same strategy as for the dip. If you don't have the assist machine, stand on a box and use your legs to provide a slight boost to pull yourself up. Then control yourself all the way down.
Bench Press for Reps: Use a weight that is three-fourths your bodyweight.
Deadlift for Reps: Use a weight that is three-fourths your bodyweight.
1-Mile Run/Walk: No modification necessary.

Although these modifications may be necessary for purposes of comparison between men and women, the goal for women should be to do everything that men can do, or do it better.

Perspective

Measures of fitness can be identified and assessed. Everyone should assess themselves and act on the results. I firmly believe that you can improve your fitness, but it is important to know where you started and then to measure your progress over time. The measures presented here are not an all-inclusive list. Don't neglect advice from your primary care physician, for example, concerning other health assessments and/or treatments. Keep in mind, though, that you are much more than numbers on a stat sheet. And possibly the best indicator of health is how you feel. The numbers can't tell the whole story. The story is yours to create as you go.

3. AEROBIC CONDITIONING

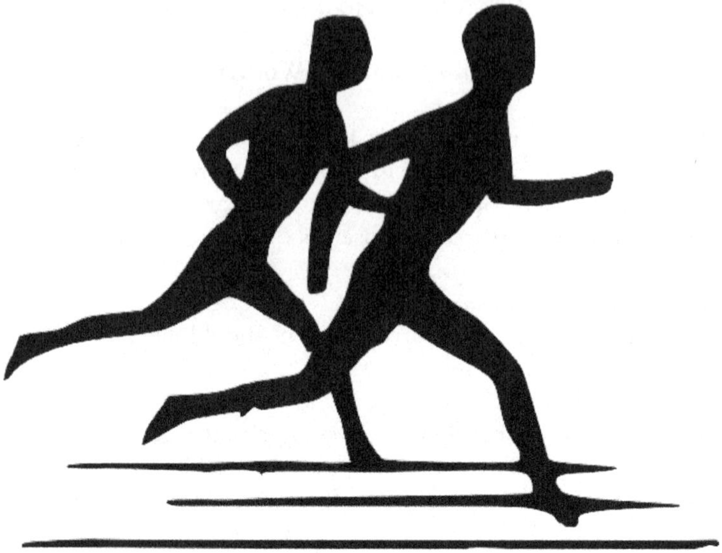

The word 'aerobics' came about when the gym instructors got together and said, "If we're going to charge $10 an hour, we can't call it jumping up and down." – Rita Rudner

The Good

Aerobic exercise – commonly called "cardio" – usually consists of running, walking, cycling, or various machines like ellipticals and steppers. Aerobic exercise conditions the heart and circulatory system. Because it requires constant movement, this form of exercise can burn a lot of calories in a relatively short period of time. For this reason many people consider aerobic exercise as the best bet for weight loss. Whether this claim is actually true or not, though, is highly debatable. The chart below lists the number of calories burned per hour of exercise.

Activity	Individual Weight and Total Calories Burned Per Hour of Exercise		
	160 lbs.	200 lbs.	240 lbs.
Aerobics, high-impact	533	664	796
Aerobics, low-impact	365	455	545
Aerobics, water	402	501	600
Basketball game	584	728	872
Bicycling, 10 mph	292	364	436
Golfing, carrying clubs	314	391	469
Hiking	438	546	654
Resistance Training	365	455	545
Rollerblading	548	683	818
Rope Jumping	861	1,074	1,286
Running, 5 mph	606	755	905
Running, 8 mph	861	1,074	1,286
Skiing, cross country	496	619	741
Swimming, laps	423	528	632
Tennis, singles	584	728	872
Walking, 3.5 mph	314	391	469

The traditional recommendation for effective aerobic exercise is to sustain an elevated heart rate for at least 20 minutes. The sustained heart rate (target) one shoots for is determined by the following formula: (220 – age)70 percent. Where 220 represents the maximum heart rate minus one's age x .7. So, taking myself as an example 220 – 50 = 170 (This is considered my maximum heart rate) x .7 = 119. This is supposed to be my target heart rate for effective cardio training. This is why most cardio machines monitor your pulse rate and give feedback as to where trainees are on the cardio scale.

To be honest, I don't pay much attention to my heart rate while training. I pay more attention to my resting heart rate, a prime indicator of fitness, with lower being better. After training for a while, you can tell how hard you are working by how heavy you are breathing. But to effectively condition your cardiovascular system, you must elevate your heart rate for periods of time, regardless of the type of exercise. I prefer a more steady state type of cardio, like walking on an incline, where I gradually increase the pace and incline up to a point where my heart rate is sufficiently elevated for 10 to 15 minutes. I also like the elliptical because I can quickly ramp up the intensity by simply moving faster. I'll move as fast as I can for a minute, then slow down for a couple of minutes. This adds variety and challenge to my cardio workouts, which helps break up the monotony.

One's weight contributes to calories burned because more weight requires more energy to move it through space. This is why most of these high-tech cardio machines ask you how much you weigh when entering your workout information. Think about how difficult it is to carry a 20 or 30 pound weight very far. You don't have to go very far before you begin to really feel that extra burden you are carrying. Relate that to how much harder your body has to work to carry around 20 to 30 pounds of fat, whenever and wherever you go. Don't put too much faith, though, on how accurate these machines count the calories you are burning. From my experience, many machines (especially the ellipticals) overestimate how many calories you use, while others (like most treadmills) underestimate the number.

I've also noticed that people tend to overestimate how many calories they are burning through exercise. On average, walking a mile burns only about 120 calories. A typical donut has about 300 calories. In this respect, one could argue that exercise is a bit overrated for the purpose of weight loss. This is not to say that exercise is futile. It does, however, underscore the fact that in order to lose and maintain your weight, you can't rely on exercise alone. Calories matter.

To put a significant dent in your caloric expenditure via exercise, you really have to ramp up your movement and do it for a considerable amount of time. Take walking again as an example. If you walk for an hour at an average of 3.5 mph, you'll end up burning around 350-400 calories or more, depending on your weight. At that rate you are starting to make a significant dent in your caloric expenditure. Look at the total calories burned by running 8 mph for an hour (1,074 for a 200-lb individual). If you can keep up this pace, you can burn some serious calories. That's one reason why most long-distance runners are slim. Not surprising, though, overweight individuals have a much harder time running, due to the extra weight they are carrying. Walking is a better option for many overweight individuals.

The Bad

While aerobic exercise is a must for every training program, you can do too much. Once again, the general principle of necessity applies: only do that which is necessary to reach your fitness goals and no more. In fact, doing more than is necessary can be very detrimental, not only to reaching your fitness goals, but to your overall health as well. In fact, extreme endurance events, like marathons, have shown to be damaging to the heart. Studies show that scar tissue can develop in the heart of extreme endurance athletes and that they are five times more likely to experience arterial fibrillation, or fluctuations in the heartbeat that can trigger more serious heart problems. Moreover, many endurance athletes don't look very healthy. They often appear gaunt and don't have much muscle mass. I believe this unhealthy appearance is due to the fact that they are so grossly over-trained. The body simply cannot sufficiently repair itself from this extensive amount of training, and therefore gets behind, which causes several of the body's systems to suffer and slowly decline.

Problems Associated With Too Much Cardio Exercise

- Can be very hard on the feet, knees, lower back and other body parts.
- Inevitably results in overtraining due to too much exercise during a particular period of time.
- Quite monotonous – hard for people to do for very long at a time.
- Can impair muscle growth because, due to the SAID principle, muscle tissue adapts to the demands placed upon it.
- Can contribute to muscle catabolism when dieting. This is due to the fact that when calories are being restricted and energy supplies are low, the body will begin utilizing amino acids from your muscles for energy. This is why most people lose at least some muscle while dieting.
- Cardio exercise does little or nothing to slow sarcopenia, the gradual loss of muscle as we age. That takes resistance exercise.
- Cardio exercise can increase appetite, which can cancel out any fat loss due to exercise.

How Cardio Exercise Interferes With Muscular Hypertrophy

There are a few important things going on here. First, cardio exercise, especially high intensity cardio, burns a lot of calories, calories that could be used to repair and build new muscle. This is an especially important consideration for the ectomorphic body type, who has trouble gaining weight in the first place. For the hard gainer, every calorie counts, and thus, if muscular hypertrophy is the primary goal, then cardio should be of low intensity and kept to a minimum amount of time.

The second thing, and no less important, is the SAID principle: Specific Adaptation to Imposed Demands. The body has remarkable abilities to adapt to exercise, but resistance and cardio exercise represent opposite ends of the exercise spectrum, which means that by doing both, you're asking the body to adapt to two divergent activities. We all have differing ratios of slow-twitch to fast-twitch muscle fibers. Slow-twitch fibers are better suited for endurance exercise and fast-twitch for speed/power movements. A marathoner has a higher proportion of slow-twitch fibers, while a sprinter has a higher proportion of fast-twitch. A higher proportion of fast-twitch fibers is associated with greater muscular strength and hypertrophy. The good news, for those trying to build more muscle, is that slow-twitch fibers can be converted into fast-twitch, by engaging in high-intensity resistance training. More endurance exercise only contributes to slow-twitch fibers remaining slow-twitch. Look at the extremes in athletes, for example: the bodybuilder, who specializes in brief, high-intensity resistance training versus the marathon runner, who specializes in long-distance running several days a week. While it's true that these diverse athletes have vastly different muscle fiber proportions to begin with, still their specific training regimens contribute greatly to the type of physique they have.

Finally, it is thought that the mechanism for cardio interference resides in the mTOR pathway, a complicated metabolic process which is necessary for muscular hypertrophy. High-intensity weightlifting enables the mTOR mechanism, while high-intensity cardio attenuates it. Low-intensity exercise, like walking, for example, probably won't hurt your muscle-building efforts. And, some moderate cardio is necessary to fully condition the cardiovascular system, which will contribute to greater performance in high-intensity weightlifting. So, the general rule is to engage in some cardio for health and performance enhancement, but keep high-intensity cardio sessions relatively brief and infrequent. It's also important not to do cardio and resistance work in the same exercise session. If possible, separate them with sufficient time, like morning and evening, or better yet, do them on separate days.

My Recommendations for Effective Cardio

- To build and maintain good cardiovascular fitness, my general recommendation is for everyone to engage in at least three cardio sessions a week, with each session lasting at least 15 minutes while maintaining, at a minimum, a pulse rate at 60 percent of one's maximum heart rate. You don't have to wear a heart monitor; after a while you will be able to determine your effective training zone. And you should challenge yourself periodically by ramping up your speed for a minute or two at a time interspersed with periods of lower intensity.
- Although any activity can be cardio in nature, I advocate activities/machines that are designed for efficiency. Therefore, I recommend jogging (either outside or on a treadmill), power walking, cycling, stepping, or elliptical machine. Many of the

machines nowadays allow you to monitor your pulse rate and total calories burned. To avoid monotony, I like to go from machine to machine during my cardio workouts. I like variety.

- Typically, if you are trying to lose weight, you need to do more cardio, simply to burn more calories. Of course, people trying to lose weight should engage in more activity, of every sort, period. For those trying to lose weight/fat, I recommend at least 4 cardio sessions a week, with each lasting a minimum of 20 minutes, and in addition to 3 to 4 resistance-training sessions.
- Your individual goals determine how much cardio you should do above the baseline amount I described above. Obviously, if you are trying to lose fat, you should do more cardio, simply to burn more calories. If you are trying to gain weight, any more cardio above baseline will only impede your efforts to gain muscle/weight.
- I recommend no more than 5 cardio sessions a week, even for those wanting to lose weight. One could, however, increase the time of each session, with 60 minutes being the maximum amount of time for any one session.
- One can and should vary the intensity of their cardio sessions. Beyond the minimum of 60 percent of maximum heart rate for 15 minutes, you should push yourself to do more work (burn more calories) in the same period of time. Challenge yourself by walking hills, for example. That will get your heart rate up in a hurry. Another way to ramp up intensity is to push yourself to the max for a brief period of time, say a minute or so, and then back off the intensity for a minute or so, and continue to repeat this cycle for the duration of your workout. If you are used to walking, for instance, you could begin walking, and then jog, run, or even sprint for a brief period and then return to walking. Keep alternating like this for the duration of your workout.
- Don't do more than is necessary to achieve your goals, and that can vary quite a bit, depending on the person and individual goals.

Perspective

- Aerobic exercise (cardio) is an efficient means of conditioning the cardiovascular system. This will result in a lower resting heart rate (RHR), which is a widely recognized indicator of high-level fitness.
- It's still debatable which method of cardio is best – high intensity intervals (HIIT) or maintaining a relatively constant pace (steady state).
- HIIT can burn a lot calories in shorter amount of time, but it's

much more demanding. Steady state burns fewer calories within the same time period but can be done for longer periods of time, and most people can at least do it.

- There is no clear-cut distinction between exercise that is strictly cardio and that which is strictly resistance. High-rep weightlifting, for instance, can be an effective cardio workout. Time is the primary concern. How long can exercise be maintained, and at what pace? Performing circuits – several resistance exercises performed without rest – can elevate and maintain your heart rate at a level to be considered effective cardio.
- While some cardio is beneficial, too much is detrimental.
- Too much cardio interferes with muscular hypertrophy.
- Too much cardio, especially at intense levels, has been shown to be damaging to the heart.
- Keep in mind that, although cardio does burn a lot of calories, it still might be a bit overrated as a primary means of losing fat. Research has shown, for example, that more exercise in general tends to stimulate appetite, thus making people eat more to make up for the energy lost due to increased exercise. It's better to look at exercise as a means to control one's weight after an ideal weight has been reached.

4. THE SCIENCE OF MUSCLE

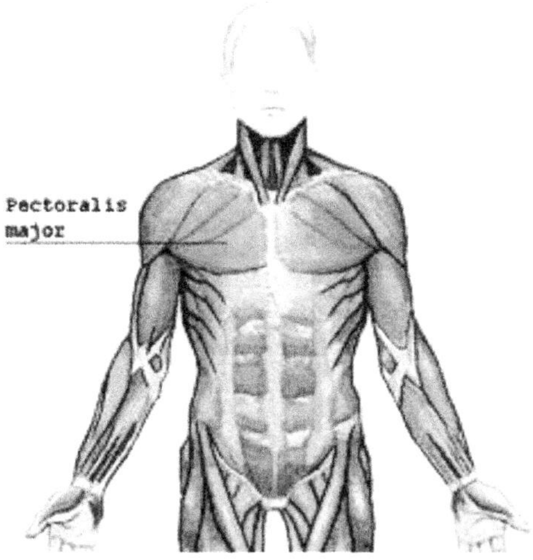

Fitness – if it came in a bottle, everybody would have a great body.
– Cher

General Training Principles

I have argued that building muscle should be the primary goal of any fitness program. With building muscle being so important, it is imperative that we have at least a basic understanding of how muscles grow.

Hypertrophy refers to gains in muscle mass, while atrophy refers to a loss of muscle. How do muscles become bigger and stronger? Skeletal muscle is the most adaptable tissue in the human body, and it is able to adapt very quickly to demands placed on it through proper training protocols. For resistance exercise, like weightlifting, to be effective, it must challenge your current strength levels. If the weight (stress) applied to the muscle is greater than it is used to, individual muscle fibers are damaged. The body responds to this stress quickly to repair the damage and put back a little more to ensure the affected muscles can handle this stress in the future. It's actually a survival mechanism much like the tanning process when the skin is exposed to sunlight.

In response to high levels of stress, cells surrounding the damaged muscle cells – called satellite cells – are recruited to bond with the damaged cells and thus help repair the damaged cells and make them slightly bigger and stronger. Growth factors are released and play an important role in tissue repair by initiating the response made by satellite cells. Insulin-like growth factor (IGF-I &II) promotes changes in the DNA of muscle cells that turns on protein synthesis. Insulin shuttles glucose and amino acids into muscle cells and also acts positively on protein synthesis. Testosterone is the primary hormone that activates protein synthesis at the cellular level.

Researchers have identified two types of hypertrophy impacting muscle cells.

1) **Sarcoplasmic Hypertrophy**: An increase in the size of muscle cells due to increased fluid volume within the muscle cells. It is speculated that an increase in sarcoplasmic hypertrophy contributes to myofibrillar hypertrophy.
2) **Myofibrillar Hypertrophy**: An increase in the size of individual muscle fibers due to an increase in contractile proteins. This growth is the net result from increased protein synthesis.

Core Training Principles

There are a myriad of training philosophies and methods, but there are only a handful of scientifically-established training principles. These core principles apply to everyone wanting to build more muscle and become more fit:

- **Progressive Overload Principle**: You must overload your muscles with increasingly greater stress to force them to adapt and grow. This is usually done by gradually increasing the weight lifted on exercises, increasing the number of sets (to a point), or decreasing the rest time between sets (to a point). Too little rest limits the amount of weight you can use and thus decreases the intensity of your workout, making it more difficult to build muscle.
- **S.A.I.D. Principle**: **S**pecific **A**daptation to **I**mposed **D**emands. In short, the body, especially your muscles, adapt in direct relation to the demands you place on them. Muscles, for example, adapt differently to lifting heavy weights than they do to running or cycling. When trying to build muscle, lifting heavy weights repetitively is going to produce greater results than any other type of exercise.
- **Principle of Transfer**: Engaging in one activity or exercise helps or transfers to a different activity or exercise. Doing leg presses may help one squat more weight or vice versa, for example. Both exercises contribute to greater muscular development of the legs. It's common for athletes to incorporate exercises into their training programs that, in theory, help them perform better in the sport

they play. Even common trainees do specific exercises to help them perform everyday tasks more efficiently. The degree of transfer increases as the similarity between the two exercises, or the exercise and the desired skill or activity, increases.

- **Specificity of Training**: Seemingly contradictory of the principle of transfer, if you want to improve in a specific activity, you should engage in that particular activity. Specificity of training always trumps transfer of training. If you want to be able to perform more pushups, for example, nothing beats doing pushups. If you want to squat a lot of weight, doing heavy leg presses will only take you so far. To reach your potential in the squat, you will have to do plenty of heavy squat sessions.
- **F.I.T.T. Principle**: **F**requency, **I**ntensity, **T**ype, and **T**ime. Four key variables in any fitness program. Briefly, frequency is how often you train; intensity is how hard you train; type is the type of training you do; and time is how long your training sessions last.
- **Holistic Training Principle**: A broad-based approach that encourages one to engage in a variety of exercises and training practices. Some people mistakenly believe that they can reach their fitness potential by engaging in only one exercise or activity, like walking, for example, or playing a sport. It's true that you can increase your fitness level by simply doing something, but to reach your potential, you must follow a comprehensive plan. As I've stated many times by now, resistance exercise should form the basis of any fitness program.

Other Considerations

- **The Law of Diminishing Returns**: This principle contains two important parts: 1) The idea that while you must train intensely to make progress, too much intense training becomes detrimental. Exactly where or when someone goes from just the right amount of training to too much training varies from one person another. My advice for everyone is to manage training intensity by limiting highly-intense workouts to no more than four days a week. 2) The second part of this principle deals with training longevity and continued results over time. It's commonly accepted that beginners to training experience the greatest results. The generally accepted reason for this is that the muscles and other systems of newbies have not been exposed to this level of training and thus are able to adapt more efficiently to the demands placed on them. It's important to remember here that adaptation to stimuli, of any sort, is a survival mechanism of the body. The longer you train, the less your body responds to your efforts. It's as if your body says, "I've seen that before, no big deal, no need to change." Why can't we simply train harder and thus continue to place new demands on our muscles? That's problematic for a couple of reasons. First, there's a limit to how hard you can train, and if you train too intensely for too long, you're bound to overtrain and stunt, or even reverse, your progress. Second, you can only get so strong and train intensely for so long until your body begins to break down. Even if you are fortunate enough to avoid major injury, micro-injuries and plain wear and tear build up over time and can negatively impact further progress. The good news is that muscle mass built over time can be maintained with a lot less training and intensity it took to build it in the first place.

- **Muscle Memory**: It's common knowledge that one can regain lost muscle much faster than it was built in the first place. There are many well-documented cases (see Colorado Experiment) of individuals regaining as much as 40 or more pounds of muscle in a matter of a few weeks, muscle that took years to build initially. It is thought that a couple of things are going on here. First, upon retraining, the neural pathways from the brain to the muscles are already in place. It's sort of like learning to ride a bike; you never forget how. And then in the initial hypertrophy process, muscles grow by laying down new proteins to make the individual fibers larger and by muscle cells incorporating nearby satellite cells into their nuclei. Now, muscles atrophy due to a decrease in the proteins that make up muscle fibers, but the larger nuclei are still there. Upon resuming intense training, protein synthesis goes back into high gear, and you are already more than half-way there.
- **Muscle Confusion**: This is a concept that is used and misused in much of the conversation surrounding fitness today. It's at the core of the most popular exercise programs out there and the common practice of periodization. Basically, it's the idea that you need to constantly change your exercises, reps, and routine in order to keep your muscles confused and thus force them to adapt to new stimuli. There is some truth to this. Forcing your muscles to adapt is what it's all about, but what is the best, or most efficient, way to accomplish this? I don't think it's necessary to continually alter your workouts, as long as your regular workouts have sufficient variety. By variety, I'm referring to doing enough exercises and switching them up on a regular basis. I'm also referring to rep ranges and the amount of weight used. All of these things can be manipulated on a regular basis, but keep in mind that some exercises are more productive than others, as well as certain rep

and weight schemes. Most experts who study muscle hypertrophy identify about 5-10 basic compound exercises that are most effective in promoting hypertrophy. Similarly, we know from years of research, as well as tons of anecdotal evidence from bodybuilders, that the most effective rep and weight scheme for building muscle is 8-12 reps at 70-80 percent of maximum weight. While muscle confusion can be utilized to some degree to help encourage muscles to adapt, the most important requirement for muscular hypertrophy is progressive overload.

Why Gaining Muscle Is So Difficult

It always amazes me when women say that they would lift weights but they don't want to build big, bulky muscles. This should be the furthest thing from their minds. For goodness sake, most men I know can't gain any muscle, even those that train consistently and hard. Women just don't produce enough testosterone to build a lot of muscle. Female bodybuilders who have big muscles are greatly supplementing their testosterone levels. Many competitive male bodybuilders, among other athletes, are supplementing their levels, too. Besides taking anabolic steroids, top-level bodybuilders have a genetic advantage over the average lifter. Some people simply have greater potential for putting on muscle, and a very few individuals are just freaks. The individual potential to add muscle is distributed normally on the bell curve, like height and intelligence, for examples. Most people are average; some are above or below average; and a few are well above or below average. For those on the low end of the continuum, gaining muscle is extremely difficult, and in some cases, virtually impossible. I have witnessed many guys train for years without gaining any appreciable muscle. This is not to say that they are not benefitting from their training. There are a myriad of beneficial effects derived from vigorous exercise, most of which being more important than the size of our muscles.

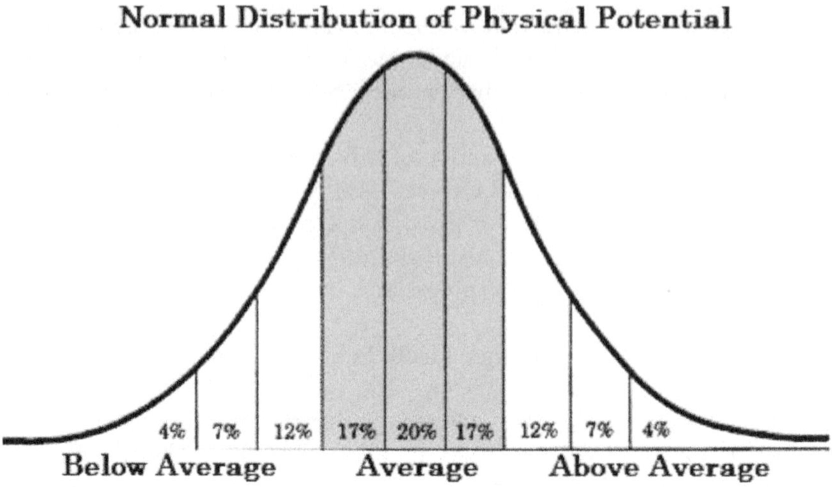

According to the Bell Curve chart above, the potential to build muscle is distributed normally within the general population. Over 50 percent of the population has average potential. You see evidence of this in gyms everywhere. Most people can make significant progress, if they train hard, eat right, and get enough rest. Those in the above-average category make gains relatively easy, while those below average see little in the way of results.

How much muscle can one expect to gain over, let's say, two years of serious training and following a sensible program, like the ones I recommend? It's often difficult to determine one's potential for gaining muscle until one actually engages in serious training. However, after a few months of training, one usually knows what his potential is. Those who have above average potential typically see gains right from the start, and those who don't, well, don't.

One common way to gauge potential is to determine your body type: ectomorph, endomorph, or mesomorph. Ectomorphs tend to be thin, lanky and have a harder time gaining weight. Endomorphs are the opposite of ectomorphs. They tend to be thicker and have a harder time losing weight. Mesomorphs tend to have the best of the other types. They tend to be lean, muscular, and athletic. Very few individuals are strictly one body type. Rather, we are combinations of two. I, for example, am somewhere between endomorph and mesomorph, since I have characteristics of both. Obviously, the more mesomorphic you are the higher your potential for gaining muscle is. Probably 95 percent of successful competitive bodybuilders are primarily mesomorphic. The problem with being too ectomorphic is that you have difficulty in gaining weight and/or muscle. Ectomorphs, then, should eat consistently and avoid extra exercise. They can get away with eating whatever and how much they want. On the contrary, the problem with being too endomorphic is that you have difficulty in losing fat. Therefore, endomorphs must constantly watch their diet and endeavor to burn as many calories as possible.

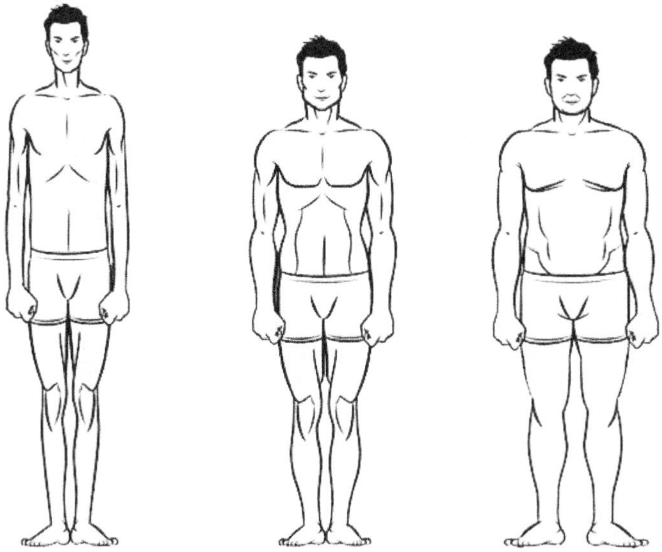

Ectomorph Mesomorph Endomorph

As a species, humans may not be genetically predisposed to have big muscles. If you consider how humans evolved, bulky muscles may have been more of a liability than a benefit. Early hunters and warriors needed strength, but agility and speed would have been more important in hunting prey or running away from predators, and extra muscle would have slowed them down. And just think how big and tasty, lean muscles would have appeared to hungry carnivores. There's no good reason to make oneself more tempting to predators that already want to eat you. Probably the biggest reason that natural selection did not favor large muscle mass is the energy requirements, in the form of food, to maintain it. When food is scarce, survival is more important than building and maintaining big muscles.

What's the Best Way to Gain Muscle?

If we could give every individual the right amount of nourishment and exercise, not too little and not too much, we would have found the safest way to health. – Hippocrates

One's potential for gaining muscle lies somewhere on a continuum, with most people somewhere in the average range, really gifted individuals on the upper end, and the muscularly-challenged on the lower end. Of course, if you are lucky enough to be on the upper end, you probably already know that you are gifted, and thus probably don't need my advice, or anyone else's for that matter. My advice is for everyone else, since everyone can make improvements to their physique, some even quite stunning. While it's true that most males predominantly want to get bigger while most women want to get smaller, that doesn't mean that men and women's training regimens should differ very much at all.

The biggest mistake I see people making in the gym is simply not training hard enough. Intense training is the core of any muscle-building program. Some exercises are better than others, but I don't see people doing the real hard lifts, like squats and deadlifts. Heck, a lot of people don't even train their legs at all. It's the training that sets the stage for your muscles to adapt to greater demands imposed upon them. I sweat quite a bit during my workouts, even in cooler, less humid weather. But, I don't see many people sweating during their workouts, which indicates that they are not working hard enough. In most cases, people train much too slowly. They do a set and then chat for ten minutes, and the set wasn't very hard to begin with. Another misdirected, albeit well-intentioned, gym practice is group training. Having a training partner for support and spotting is fine, but when you get more than three training together, there's more resting than training. And then guys have this distorted method of "spotting" one another where it is difficult to tell which one is actually doing the set and which one is spotting. I don't know how many times I see a guy doing a bench press and his spotter basically doing a deadlift. Guys, let's go a little easier on the spotting. Make the lifter do most of the work. I actually like to train alone. If I need a spot – which isn't that often – I just ask someone, and I don't work them to death.

Some think that nutrition is something like 90 percent of the muscle-building process, but I believe that is a major overstatement. Training is far more important than nutrition. Obviously, nutrition is important. You must fuel your body for maximum performance, which means meeting, and exceeding to some extent, your body's requirement for macro and micro nutrients. In order to put yourself in a muscle-building (anabolic) state, you must consume more calories than you expend. To build muscle, the energy must come from somewhere. Many guys have trouble gaining weight. You simply have to keep the calories coming all day long. In some ways, these individuals have it good; they can eat literally whatever they want and how much they want without gaining much, if any, fat. Of course, they also have trouble putting on muscle, too.

While weight training theories abound, there are a few core principles that should be adhered to for optimal progress:

- **Progressive Overload**: Muscles will adapt to greater demands placed upon them. To overload the muscles, one must lift more weight, perform more reps with same amount of weight, or rest less between sets.
- The best **Rep Range** for gaining muscle is 8-12, using about 70-80 percent of your one-rep max. Fewer than 6 reps emphasizes strength and power. That's why powerlifters train with very heavy weight and low reps; they are only concerned with lifting a maximum amount of weight for a single rep. More than 15 reps trains more for endurance, which can still be intense enough to stimulate hypertrophy. High rep training also burns a lot of calories and creates a good pump within the muscles trained, which contributes to sarcoplasmic hypertrophy.
- **Time Under Tension**: The amount of time a set lasts, or the total time resistance is applied, should be between 40 and 60 seconds. So, if you do a set of 10 reps, each rep should last approximately 4 to 6 seconds. This could mean 2 seconds up and 4 seconds down. This also means that you should focus at least as much time, or more, on the negative (the lowering) portion of the rep as you spend on the positive (the raising) portion, since the negative portion has been shown to do the most damage to the targeted muscle. This is one time when being negative is a good thing.
- **Recovery**: Muscles that have been trained intensely need time to recover and rebuild. The workout merely applies the stimulus; it's during rest that muscles actually repair themselves and grow. After an intense workout, muscles require anywhere from 48 to 72 hours, and possibly longer, before they have recovered enough to be trained again. Overzealous trainees work out too often, which only stymies any potential progress.
- **Metabolic Stress**: Metabolism describes the body's process of utilizing calories, or energy. So, metabolic stress increases in proportion to the rate in which the body is burning calories. It's measured as a function of time and the relative difficulty of the exercise performed. In terms of resistance exercise, for example, metabolic stress increases if 1) the intensity of the exercise (in terms of weight and/or number of reps) is increased; and 2) rest periods between sets decrease. Therefore, it is generally accepted that the same amount of work performed in a shorter period of time increases metabolic stress and makes for a more intense and productive workout.

- **Mechanical Tension**: This refers to the actual load or weight applied to a muscle during exercise. To stimulate muscular hypertrophy, the weight needs to be in the range of 75 to 90 percent of one's 1-rep max, and the number of reps performed need to be in the range of 6 to 12. Now, this is where mechanical tension overlaps with metabolic stress, and both concepts are vital to gaining muscle. The amount of weight used is obviously important, but so is the rest time between sets. If you use too much weight and rest too long between sets, mechanical tension is increased, but at the expense of metabolic stress. On the other hand, if you rest too little and reduce weight too low, metabolic stress is enhanced at the expense of mechanical tension. As it turns out, the best relationship between the these two concepts is to rest only one to two minutes between sets while trying to keep the weight lifted between 70 and 80 percent of your max while still performing 6 to 12 reps each set. This practice accentuates both training concepts maximally.

A Note on Anabolic Steroids

Anabolic steroids, often referred to as performance-enhancing drugs, make the news quite often these days, most notably when high-profile athletes get caught using them. And from all accounts, those caught cheating represent only a small fraction of the total number using them at any one time. In other words, it seems likely that the use of anabolic steroids in professional sports is widespread, including sports that you might not expect, like cycling and golf, for examples. The same could be said for high-level amateur athletics as well.

Should we be surprised at the pervasiveness of anabolic steroids in the athletic arena? We shouldn't be. Athletes have always searched for ways to gain an edge over the competition. Athletes take all sorts of vitamins, supplements, potions, and concoctions, engage in all sorts of novel training regimens, and utilize the latest training equipment and gadgets in an effort to gain the slightest competitive edge. Well, anabolic steroids represent the ultimate competitive edge. To borrow a popular phrase, they have literally been a game changer.

Athletes aren't the only ones using anabolic steroids. According to surveys, the most common steroid users are adult males between the ages of 24 and 40. And now more males over the age of 40 are beginning to replace declining testosterone levels. Seen all the "low-T" ads lately? Men, as a whole, want to be bigger and stronger, and in some sense, more assertive and self-confident. Well, testosterone is what makes men, men.

The profound popularity and impact of anabolic steroids on our culture has been due to their ability to enhance muscle growth and recuperation.

There's no doubt that anabolic steroids can help you maximize your physical potential, but I'm going to tell you why you probably shouldn't take them.

Anabolic steroids can be extremely damaging to the body. Anytime you mess with your hormones, you're asking for trouble. Muscle cells have androgen receptors, which testosterone molecules bind to and exert their muscle-building effects by telling the cell to increase protein synthesis. The problem is that these androgen receptors are also located in other parts of the body, like the skin, heart, brain, and prostate, and testosterone does its work in these places, too, which results in many of the side effects associated with steroid use. These can include acne, an enlarged prostate, and possibly an enlarged heart. The heart is a muscle, after all. Other common side effects include high blood pressure (due to fluid retention), liver damage (especially with oral steroids), and excessive aggression.

As with all drugs, dosage is critical. There are therapeutic dosages that will, in most cases, do little harm to the body. However, in order to maximize muscle growth, users almost always exceed therapeutic dosages, and side effects are related to the dose. Another factor is the amount of time a drug is taken. Extended time on steroids, combined with high dosages, sets users (abusers) up for future health problems. And with the ultra-high dosages that many bodybuilders take, we are seeing more heart, kidney, and liver problems within the bodybuilding community.

Almost everyone assumes that anabolic steroids can turn anyone into a Hercules and that everyone who is heavily muscled must be taking them. Both assumptions are faulty. First, steroids don't work the same for everyone. Some people experience good results while taking them. Others see little results from the same dosage and similar training protocols. Side effects also vary widely from one user to the next. It's safe to say, that for high-level bodybuilders, steroids worked very well. However, keep in mind that these individuals have the best genetics for gaining muscle to begin with. I hypothesize that steroids produce greater gains in muscle for those who already have good genetics for gaining muscle, and I think this is due to fact that these genetically-gifted individuals already have more muscle cells and thus more androgen receptors, which allow steroid molecules to work their magic. So, I think that the old saying in bodybuilding circles is true. If there were no steroids at all, the top bodybuilders would still be the top bodybuilders, due primarily to their genetic advantage. Then, there are some guys and gals who, due to superlative genetics, respond very well to training, and thus put on muscle quickly. So, just because someone exhibits pronounced musculature doesn't mean that they are juicing.

Anabolic steroids are extremely expensive on the black market, and that's the only way you are going to get them. No doctor, who values his medical license, is going to prescribe them to you these days. Just 10 cc's of injectable testosterone – about a 4-5 week supply – will cost you around $200.00. And test is one of the cheaper items out there. People wanting to gain a lot of muscle – like competitive bodybuilders, for example – take a lot more than straight test. They combine several drugs as once, a practice known in bodybuilding inner circles as "shotgunning." The idea by combining drugs is that together they will create a synergistic anabolic effect. Whether the technique works or not, there's no doubt that it can be extremely expensive. Bodybuilders routinely spend over $1,000.00 on an 8-week cycle of steroids, and this doesn't take into account human growth hormone, which is now common among bodybuilders and other athletes and vastly more expensive than steroids.

On the black market there's no guarantee that what you are paying an arm and an leg for is what you are actually getting. With so much potential profit out there for these drugs, the black market is flooded with fake products. Some counterfeits may not even be sterile. It's easy enough to order these drugs through the internet, but keep in mind that they are illegal to possess or to ship through the mail. So, each time you receive an order, you are breaking the law and risk getting caught, which could result in a felony conviction and possibly imprisonment.

In short, anabolic steroids are illegal and therefore may get you in trouble with the law. Buying them on the black market, you are never absolutely certain that what you are getting is the real thing, that they contain the proper potency, or that they are even safe for human consumption. Steroids are extremely expensive, especially considering that what you buy might not even be the real thing. Finally, steroids can be potentially dangerous to your long-term health, and they might not even work as well as you think they will. So, consider these points before you ever try steroids. In my view, for the average person just wanting to put on some muscle, the cons far outweigh the pros. Work hard, eat right, take the proper supplements, and see what you can accomplish. You might actually surprise yourself.

Now, I must admit that my perspective changes a little when considering the same decision for professional athletes, or others than can make money or earn fame due to their athletic prowess. I'm certainly not advising anyone to take steroids, but I can certainly understand why professional athletes do so. Whoever you are, if you do decide to take steroids, by all means do your research on the drug's effects on the body (good and bad). Work with your physician if you can and especially monitor your blood work and blood pressure. Take the minimum dosage and only for a few weeks at a time. In other words, be smart and proactive about your health.

5. APPROACHES TO TRAINING

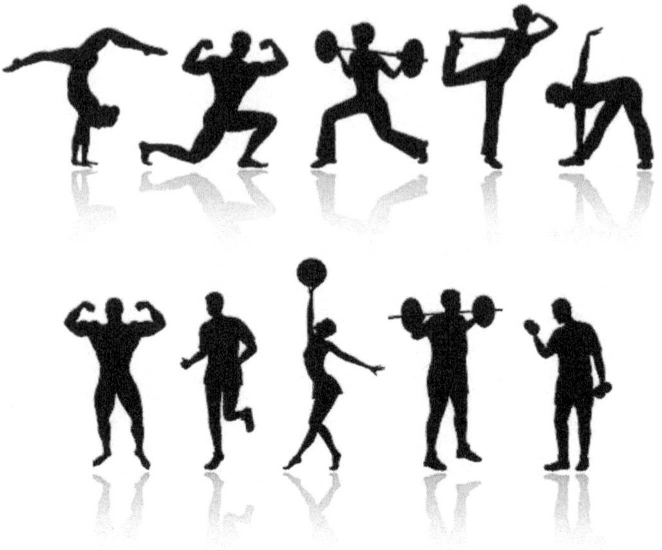

What fits your busy schedule better, exercising one hour a day or being dead 24 hours a day? – Randy Glasbergen

In over 30 years of working out, I've tried just about every conceivable training approach or method out there. I've lifted weights, run thousands of miles, and played several sports. There are many approaches to enhancing fitness, and some have such dedicated followers to the point that they can rightly be called subcultures. People have different goals. Many people who exercise on a regular basis participate in more than one activity, like aerobics and yoga, as examples. Others tend to specialize, as in the case of a marathon runner or bodybuilder. It's widely recognized that to perform at a high level, to be competitive, or to maximize one's potential, one must devote a considerable amount of time to that activity. This devotion leaves little time for other activities. And in such disparate activities as endurance running versus bodybuilding, one has to specialize on one or the other, since one activity interferes with the other to some extent – not only in terms of time but performance as well.

Are some activities better than others in promoting fitness, and, if so, what kind of metrics can we use to rate and compare activities? Keep in mind that any exercise is better than no exercise, and any exercise regimen is better than sporadic exercise. My intent here is to review the most common approaches to training, including their relative pros and cons and to apply my own rating scale to each one. Here I describe the most common approaches to training by using the name corresponding to the devotee of the approach.

My rating scale consists of the two performance-related areas most commonly associated with fitness (muscular hypertrophy and cardiovascular conditioning), along with the accessibility of performing and participating in the activity, and the relative cost. My rating scale weights muscular hypertrophy more heavily than the other variables, due to its importance in promoting fitness.

You might think that my rating criteria are rather narrow, but keep in mind that I'm looking at the variables that we have the most control over – cardiovascular endurance and muscular strength and size. One could argue for other measures, like agility, balance, speed, and others. There's a couple of problems, though, with doing this. First, the variables I just mentioned are difficult to measure easily. Cardiovascular endurance and muscular strength and size are relatively easy to measure. Second, those other variables fall more into the category of skill and thus are generally associated with sports or athletic performance. If you participate in a specific sport, then you know what it's like to work on sharpening those skills that will help you to perform better. I'm certainly not against anybody spending time on developing specific athletic skills, as doing so involves much exercise and conditioning. I'm simply arguing that, for the vast majority of the population, trying to improve cardiovascular endurance and muscular strength and size are by far the easiest, as well as most productive, ways to enhance fitness.

Here are the variables I rated and the total points I have assigned to each:

- **Muscular Hypertrophy**: How effective the approach is in promoting muscle growth. Maximum Points: 10
- **Cardiovascular Conditioning**: How effective the approach is in conditioning the cardiovascular system. Maximum Points: 8
- **Accessibility**: How easy it is for one to participate in the activity. Some activities require specialized skills, equipment, and/or facilities. Maximum Points: 5
- **Cost**: How affordable is the activity? Maximum Points: 5

This gives a maximum score of 28.

Movers and Shakers

This group consists primarily of those who participate in aerobics-type classes, such as step aerobics or zumba. As discussed in Chapter 3, aerobic exercise typically consists of low-intensity, repetitive movement that can be done for relatively long periods of time, such as running or cycling. These types of classes have been hugely popular, especially among women, who, more so than men, tend to want to exercise in groups. Participants move, hop, step and stretch for about an hour per session. It's a relatively effective workout for getting the heart rate elevated for an extended period of time and burning a significant number of calories. The problem is that many who participate in aerobics do no other type of exercise, like resistance work, for example. If you are doing aerobics but no serious resistance work, then you are getting only half a workout and half the benefit of what most gyms have to offer. Aerobics can help you lose weight, since you do burn a lot of calories in one session. However, you have to lift weights in order to build muscle and get that "toned" look that so many desire. Unfortunately, many women still think that lifting weights will bulk them up, but this is simply not true.

Muscular Hypertrophy	Endurance/ Conditioning	Accessibility	Cost	Total
2	6	3	3	14

Pros: Provides a decent cardio workout; is relatively inexpensive; and is reasonably accessible, since most gyms offer classes and you need little equipment.
Cons: Very little resistance work for building muscle; have to attend when classes are offered.

Runners

With runners, I am referring to all long-distance type activities, like marathon running, cycling, or triathlons. Running is simply the most popular endurance activity. It seems as though everyone wants to do a marathon these days. Endurance events are aerobics taken to the extreme. Runners preparing for a marathon can run anywhere from 50 to 100 miles a week. And that's my problem with endurance training; it creates a state of severe overtraining in the body. Exercise is good, but too much exercise can be unhealthy. Endurance athletes don't look healthy. They do have low bodyfat, but they have little muscle mass as well. They often have a gaunt look, like they've been starving themselves. Even more so than the aerobics group, endurance trainers place all their emphasis on endurance and little, if any, energy on anything else. Well, how could they? They already spend way too much time running. Endurance athletes are in desperate need of resistance work, but to do that, they first need to drastically reduce their volume of endurance work.

Muscular Hypertrophy	Endurance/ Conditioning	Accessibility	Cost	Total
1	8	2	5	16

Pros: Best method for cardio conditioning; low cost – just good shoes.
Cons: Provides little or no hypertrophy training; many people simply can't run and probably shouldn't; many runners develop chronic injuries.

Walkers

Walking is, arguably, the most popular form of exercise on the planet. The treadmill is still the most popular piece of equipment at the gym. Walkers enjoy the simplicity of walking, putting one foot in front of the other. Walking is, after all, something that most people can do, and, contrary to other forms of exercise, can enjoy doing it. There's nothing like a peaceful stroll or hike with beautiful scenery to clear the mind and commune with nature. Therefore, walking may be the single best exercise one can do. Walking can be an effective form of aerobic training, especially if you walk at a brisk pace and incorporate hills into your route. One problem is that many walkers don't walk at a pace that challenges their cardiovascular system. And you don't burn as many calories walking as you might think. Walking a mile burns only about 120 calories on average. I enjoy walking outside, as it always seems to go by faster than walking on a treadmill. However, I recommend investing in a treadmill so weather is no longer a factor. Then, there's no excuse to not walk.

Muscular Hypertrophy	Endurance/ Conditioning	Accessibility	Cost	Total
1	4	5	5	15

Pros: Is the most accessible and affordable fitness activity; can provide a high degree of cardio conditioning, if hills are incorporated.
Cons: Virtually no muscular hypertrophy, and not the best cardio conditioning, either.

Karate Kids

The martial arts originated in China over 4,000 years ago as, primarily, a means of self-defense. Karate classes, as well as the other martial arts, gained popularity in the U.S. during the early 70s due in large part to Bruce Lee's martial arts fight scenes on the big screen. Since then, the martial arts have become part of our popular culture. Who can forget *The Karate Kid*? Big time action stars like Chuck Norris, Jackie Chan, Jean-Claude van Damme, and Steven Seagal have taken the martial arts in film to epic levels. Now, nearly all fight scenes contain some elements of the martial arts.

Martial arts classes have seen periods of huge popularity through the years. The attainment of higher degrees of skill – in the color of belts – serves as motivation to participants. "Black belt" is one of the most recognizable terms in our modern lexicon. Students also have the opportunity to compete in regional, state, and national competitions. Martial arts classes stress self-discipline as much as physical fitness or technical skill. Kick boxing has shown up in aerobic-type classes, either on its own or part of a larger system, like Tae Bo. In recent years, mixed martial arts (MMA) training sessions have shown up in gyms and dojos due to the rising popularity of MMA fighting competitions. It's interesting, though, that MMA fights look nothing like the martial arts sequences depicted in the movies. Movie fight scenes are mainly punches and kicks, whereas MMA matches are primarily grappling. I guess that two dudes holding each other on the floor is not as exciting as sweeping kicks and karate chops.

Muscular Hypertrophy	Endurance/ Conditioning	Accessibility	Cost	Total
3	3	4	4	14

Pros: Classes can be enjoyable and challenging; a variety of exercises and movements are performed, which targets flexibility, balance, endurance, and power; self-discipline and sportsmanship are stressed.
Cons: Not an efficient means of promoting muscular hypertrophy or cardio conditioning; can be expensive; hard to do as a solo activity; needs to be done in a class.

Casual Lifters

Casual lifters are those guys who like to lift weights but do little else to improve their fitness. I limit this category to all those people out there, mainly men, who simply like to hit the weights every now and then, either in a gym or at home. The workout regularity of this group varies quite a bit, from several days a week to several days a month. This group's MO is inconsistency. I've noticed that casual lifters will dedicate themselves to a lifting regimen for a few weeks but, inevitably, fizzle out. Some even quit lifting for a while before getting their motivation back and returning to the gym. Many casual lifters become discouraged due to lack of progress. Part of their problem is a general lack of commitment . . . to their training, nutrition, and rest. Many guys in this group don't have the best genetics for building muscle, but they could see better results, if they were more consistent.

Muscular Hypertrophy	Endurance/ Conditioning	Accessibility	Cost	Total
5	2	3	3	13

Pros: Provides some muscular hypertrophy; is relatively accessible and affordable.
Cons: Most lifters don't train intensely enough to maximize muscular or cardio conditioning.

Serious Lifters

This group consists of lifters who are concerned with hoisting the most weight possible, in a very limited number of specific lifts in structured competition. Powerlifters, for example, concentrate on just three lifts: the squat, bench press, and deadlift. The best lifts in each event are totaled together to come up with a composite score. In olympic-style lifting, lifters compete in only two lifts: the clean and press and the snatch. Unlike most common lifters, serious lifters are generally extremely committed to their training and nutrition. It is common for serious lifters to train at a gym that caters to either powerlifters or Olympic lifters. Most commercial gyms don't cater to these types of lifters, since they are known to frequently drop weights, grunt and scream, and get chalk all over the place. They also tend to bend bars, tear up the equipment, and generally make a mess. For most commercial gyms, serious lifters are more trouble than they are worth. I have seen some gyms set aside a room just for serious lifters in order to segregate them from the general populace.

Muscular Hypertrophy	Endurance/ Conditioning	Accessibility	Cost	Total
7	2	2	3	15

Pros: Promotes muscular strength and power.

Cons: Tends to neglect cardio conditioning; many gyms do not accommodate power or Olympic lifters.

Hardcore Bodybuilders

When you think of bodybuilders, some get the image of huge muscle heads posing in every mirror they encounter. While that image may be true in some cases, that doesn't mean that you shouldn't emulate their training. Bodybuilders certainly train in a way that maximizes muscle while minimizing bodyfat. What really sets bodybuilders apart from other lifters or other athletes in general is the very low levels of bodyfat they achieve in order to showcase their muscularity, and vascularity to some extent. In addition to extremely intense weight-lifting sessions, most bodybuilders also perform several cardio sessions a week to help in the burning of unwanted bodyfat. Many bodybuilders are quite strong, but lifting maximum weights is not their primary goal and isn't the best approach for muscular hypertrophy, anyway.

The bodybuilding approach relies on the scientifically established principles of muscular hypertrophy and is therefore vastly more effective and efficient than any other type of training for building muscle. In fact, bodybuilding is the only approach that has made it possible for individuals to maximize their muscular potential. And this is as true for women as it is for men. Most people mistakenly believe that competitive bodybuilders train for hours a day, every day. Some hardcore bodybuilders do train too long and too often, but keep in mind that many competitive bodybuilders naturally have greater recuperative capacities than the average person. The problem with many bodybuilders is that they enjoy training so much that they end up overtraining, or they spend so much time in the gym that they have little time for other important life pursuits, like relationships, for example.

I propose two separate categories for bodybuilders – hardcore and cerebral. Hardcore bodybuilders are separated from cerebral bodybuilders and other lifters in that their only goal is to improve their physique – to look better – by building muscle and losing fat, and to attain that physique through any means necessary. In this sense, they may be the most extreme athletes in any sport. They are as fanatical about their diet as they are their training. The problem for hardcore bodybuilders is that their goals – huge muscles and ultra-low bodyfat levels – are extremely difficult to attain, so much so that the result of pursuing them is having to put one's health in jeopardy.

Many hardcore bodybuilders compete in bodybuilding contests and most simply want to become as big and muscular as humanly possible. This pursuit of muscular size requires extreme measures in terms of training, nutrition, and supplementation. To aid in their quest for size, they often turn to anabolic steroids, human growth hormone, and a vast array of dietary supplements. I've known many bodybuilders who would literally do or ingest anything, if they thought it would help them achieve their goals.

Muscular Hypertrophy	Endurance/ Conditioning	Accessibility	Cost	Total
10	4	2	2	18

Pros: Main emphasis is on muscular hypertrophy; also stresses some cardio conditioning.
Cons: Hardcore culture often leads to overtraining and extreme training and nutritional strategies; an exaggerated emphasis on costly and questionable dietary supplements.

Cerebral Bodybuilders

I refer to myself as a bodybuilder, and for much of my life, I was hardcore, and still am to a certain extent. But something has happened over the past 10 years or so that has made me reevaluate my training and nutrition. In short, I've become older, and I hope, wiser. I've learned that the hardcore approach, while effective, is unsustainable over the course of one's life. When you get into your 40's, you start thinking about longevity, not just of your life but also your quality of life. I've learned that I can still train hard, but I needed to train smarter. This meant easing up on my joints by concentrating on feeling the weight instead of seeing how much I could lift and by utilizing machines more often.

By using "cerebral," I don't want to imply that hardcore bodybuilders don't think. Obviously, they know a great deal about training and nutrition. I am merely suggesting that they often do not see the big picture. They are blinded by a singular goal at the expense of other important life pursuits. In contrast to the extremism of hardcore bodybuilding, cerebral bodybuilding represents a more sensible approach to training and diet. By "cerebral," I'm also suggesting that bodybuilders can and should be critical thinkers. One must be able to sort through conflicting data and weigh scientific evidence instead of simply following gym lore or the training program of the month featured in a muscle magazine. I'm also describing a more balanced lifestyle, one that contributes to all facets of health and fitness, as well as allowing time for the development of other potentialities. I look at it this way: all cerebral bodybuilders are hardcore, but not all hardcore bodybuilders are cerebral.

All trainees desire a balanced, aesthetic physique, and, due to their training and nutrition practices, trainees in this group are the ones most likely to attain this physical ideal, while also optimizing health. In my opinion, this group represents the epitome of effective and balanced training. Individuals in this group engage in a proper balance of resistance and aerobic work, and they do so without overtraining. This means that their workouts are efficient and based on sound science. Some of the key characteristics of cerebral trainers include:

- A balance between training and recovery.
- A balanced, yet sensible, diet that powers intense workouts and provides all of the nutrients necessary for optimum health.
- Consistent training and sound nutritional practices applied over the course of one's life.
- A balance between pursuit of one's fitness goals and other important life goals.

While cerebral trainees often participate in a number of exercise activities – like aerobics, yoga, or an organized sport – in addition to resistance training and cardio, the bedrock of their fitness program is always resistance training. Resistance training is the best way, and really the only way, to build muscle, and the only way to maintain muscle while trying to lose fat. Resistance training can even be used for an effective cardio workout, if one reduces the weight and rest times. I encourage trainees to include targeted cardio work in their fitness programs because it is the most efficient means of conditioning the cardiovascular system and burning fat. The key to developing the most productive training program is striking the right balance between the amounts of resistance and cardio work. I discuss this in more detail in the next chapter.

Muscular Hypertrophy	Endurance/ Conditioning	Accessibility	Cost	Total
10	6	3	3	22

Pros: Promotes critical thinking, in addition to maximum fitness; develops maximum muscular hypertrophy through sensible training and nutritional strategies.
Cons: All combined, gym membership, healthful food, and effective dietary supplements can be somewhat costly.

Stretchers and Contortionists

This group consists of those who participate in primarily stretching workouts, such as yoga, and to some extent Pilates. I debated over calling what these individuals do in their sessions "workouts," since there's not much real work accomplished. I often quip that yoga is exercise for people who don't like to exercise. I mean, how much exercise is stretching? I'm not saying that these stretching sessions are easy. They're not. If you've ever participated in or witnessed a yoga class, you have seen some of the positions that participants contort their bodies into. There's evidence that yoga does have real physical and mental benefits. I'm just saying that, compared to other forms of exercise, stretching burns far fewer calories. Therefore, if you're trying to lose weight, you'll have to engage in more exercise than just stretching.

It's no surprise that yoga and Pilates classes are female dominated, not that men couldn't benefit from a little more stretching and meditation. Too many women steer clear of resistance work because they fear that it will bulk them up. So, they gravitate towards aerobics and/or yoga. While stretching can be beneficial as part of a fitness program, I believe that the value of flexibility is a bit overrated. You need to be flexible enough to perform the tasks in your work or daily activities. It doesn't take a yoga class to get you to this point. By far, people should be concentrating their efforts and time on results-producing resistance and cardio work. If you're that concerned with flexibility, do 10 toe touches every morning and evening.

Muscular Hypertrophy	Endurance/ Conditioning	Accessibility	Cost	Total
2	1	4	4	11

Pros: Is accessible and affordable for most people; has shown to improve mood and help depressed individuals.
Cons: Exercise isn't intense enough to develop muscular hypertrophy or cardio conditioning.

Cross-Trainers

These are people who work out, usually on a regular basis, but also participate in one or more sports. It's common, for example, for guys to lift weights or run two or three times a week while also playing basketball or softball two or three times a week. In some cases, guys try to use their running or lifting to help them in the sport they play. Many people in this category are in good shape, since they typically get a lot of exercise. Many are athletic or were athletes in school, and they continue to participate in sports, if at least informally.

Muscular Hypertrophy	Endurance/ Conditioning	Accessibility	Cost	Total
2	4	4	4	14

Pros: Provides a lot of exercise; has relatively high accessibility and low cost.
Cons: Workouts are often sporadic; muscular hypertrophy is not emphasized.

Crossfit

Over the past decade or so, Crossfit has exploded onto the fitness scene. Heck, "burpee" has practically become a household word. Crossfit has become so popular that it now warrants its own category, even though it attempts to cover the entire fitness spectrum. With crossfit, people do a little bit of everything . . . weight lifting, running, functional-type movements, stretching, and they do so with high intensity. Intensity is increased by always attempting to decrease the time it takes to complete a workout. There's no doubt that crossfit can enhance fitness. My problem with crossfit is not that it's intense, but that, for the average trainee, it may be too intense. It's not that it covers a broad range of exercises; it's that most of the exercises are performed without rest. For most people, it's simply too demanding to do on a long-term basis. With this, aerobic conditioning is promoted at the expense of muscular hypertrophy. In regard to crossfit, and some other training approaches, it may be effective at enhancing athletic skill and all-around fitness, but relatively ineffective at promoting muscular hypertrophy. And because of that flaw, I think it can be incorporated into your fitness program, but only as a break from your regular training, or, in other words, as a form of periodization. One could, for example, do a week's worth of crossfit one week out of the month, or one crossfit workout every fourth or fifth regular workout.

Muscular Hypertrophy	Endurance/ Conditioning	Accessibility	Cost	Total
5	7	2	2	16

Pros: Enhances fitness, provided that one is able to perform the workouts; promotes weight loss due to the high number of calories burned; enhances sports and functional skills and therefore may be well-suited for athletes; provides variety since different types of exercises are used; some people enjoy working out with a group.
Cons: Is too demanding for most people to stick with over the long term;

muscular hypertrophy is compromised due to too little rest between exercises and not producing enough intensity; crossfit can be expensive. a crossfit facility is typically more expensive than a regular commercial gym. some people put together their own crossfit gym, but that can get expensive as well.

Players

The player is the guy (almost always a guy) who plays a sport on a regular basis (usually only for fun) but who engages in no other formal exercise. Players can get a lot of exercise, or very little, depending on the sport. Basketball or volleyball is better than, say, softball. But, then again, as I've said ad nauseam, any exercise is better than no exercise. A lot of these guys incur injuries that sideline them from playing their chosen sport. And injuries often can limit other forms of exercise, even if the person wanted to get into a structured training program. Many people who play a sport for fun don't fully realize the potential benefits of a well-planned training program – for both conditioning and injury prevention. Look at the intense training programs of professional athletes, for example. I'm not suggesting that one has to go that far, but a little more emphasis on conditioning may pay off in the long run.

Muscular Hypertrophy	Endurance/ Conditioning	Accessibility	Cost	Total
1	5	4	4	14

Pros: Competition adds motivation; often provides regular cardio exercise; is relatively accessible and affordable, depending on the specific activity.
Cons: Muscular hypertrophy is neglected; some players don't "play" often enough.

Weekend Warriors

These are the guys who only exercise on the weekend, as if that's the only time you can engage in exercise. Most of the guys who do this get together with other weekend warriors and play basketball, or some other game. This weekly ritual inevitably results in very sore, or pulled, muscles on Monday, which require the rest of the week to recover.

In their defense (they typically don't play any) some guys do work long hours during the week, which can cut into exercise time in the evenings. In addition, some guys have fairly strenuous jobs and thus get quite a bit of exercise at work. Still, these guys would benefit from a more structured program, even if that meant simply doing some push-ups and jumping jacks at home two or three evenings a week.

Muscular Hypertrophy	Endurance/ Conditioning	Accessibility	Cost	Total
1	2	4	4	11

Pros: Some exercise is better than none.
Cons: Not enough exercise; too much at one time; increased risk of injury.

After rating all these training approaches, I want to stress that each of these can certainly play a role in your fitness program. I rated them only to give my opinion as to which approach is the most effective and efficient in promoting fitness. In other words, I based my ratings on how effective these methods of exercise are at producing the most gains in the least amount of time. In reality, most people who exercise on a regular basis engage in more than one of these activities. As long as you are doing some sort of exercise on regular basis, you are already doing better than much of the population. I'm much more concerned about getting non-exercisers to do something than I am about the particular type of exercise they do.

Perspective

- The most effective exercise programs focus primarily on muscular hypertrophy and secondarily on cardio conditioning.
- Access to and cost of an exercise activity are also important considerations in rating its potential to enhance fitness.
- Cerebral bodybuilding is the most effective and efficient means of achieving high-level fitness.
- If time permits, it's productive to participate in a variety of exercise activities.
- Since it's better to do some exercise than to do nothing, participate in something that you like, and you are much more likely to keep it up over time.

6. BUILDING MUSCLE

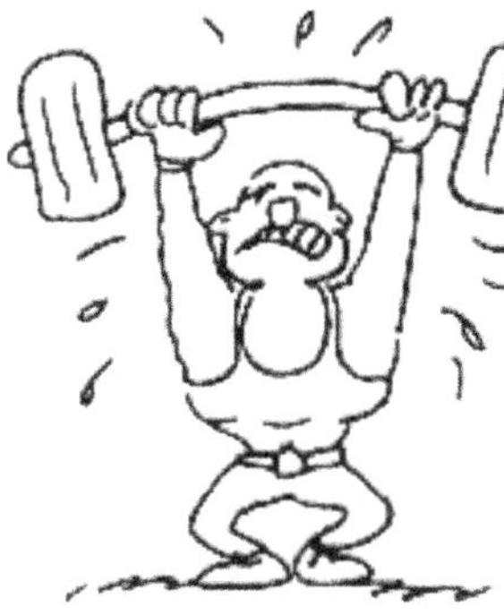

Everybody wants to be a bodybuilder, but don't nobody wanna lift no heavy ass weights – Ronnie Coleman

Being a bodybuilder myself, I advocate a training program based on intense resistance work. I can't emphasize enough the importance of intense resistance exercise, as it is the best way to build muscle, and building muscle should form the basis of any fitness-promoting program. Not everyone needs to be a bodybuilder per se, but anyone wanting to build muscle should utilize the techniques and routines common to bodybuilding. Whatever you think of bodybuilding in general, you can't argue with the fact that bodybuilders represent the pinnacle in muscular hypertrophy. In other words, bodybuilding has been shown to be the most effective program to build muscle. At the same time, however, I recognize the fitness-promoting benefits of aerobic exercise, as well as other approaches to fitness, like crossfit, for example.

The program that I detail here represents a balanced and analytical approach (the Cerebral approach), which has worked best for me over the years. It is based on the core principles of muscular hypertrophy enhancement featured in Chapter 4. Keep in mind that my program is intended to build muscle and shed bodyfat in the most efficient manner possible, all while avoiding injury. In addition to my program, I present beginning and intermediate programs. You should bear in mind that your program must be adapted to your individual fitness goals. A beginner, for example, should not follow my advanced workout, but instead should start with the beginning workout while incorporating the scientific principles that I describe.

My routine consists of three separate workouts: 1) legs (including hamstrings, lower back, glutes, and calves); 2) chest and arms; and 3) back and shoulders (including traps). Typically, I train 4 days a week, following, essentially, an every-other-day split routine. I will train two days in a row, but I don't like to train chest and arms and back and shoulders on consecutive days, due to the obvious interference in recuperation.

Below are examples of my three primary workouts. The type of set refers to how the exercise is to be performed for that particular set. A warm-up is just that, a light weight to get the muscle prepared for heavier weight. Generally, larger muscles require more warming up than smaller ones. A pyramid set is a sub-maximal performance, which is followed by a heavier set with fewer reps. A pyramid set can be thought of as an intermediate set between the warm-up and the heavier, more demanding sets. Failure means that the set is taken to failure and no more. Rest/pause means that the set is to be taken to failure and then after a short rest, additional reps are performed. I prefer a 3 to 5-second rest between rest/pause reps. A back-off set is intended to tap into more muscle fibers through higher reps and thus bring a lot of blood into the muscle. The weight to be lifted is the percent of your one-rep max in that particular lift. The amount of reps and weight are only approximations and can vary across workouts.

Workout #1, Legs		
Exercise	**Type of Set**	**Sets/Reps/Percent of Max**
Smith Machine Squats	Warm-up	1x10, 40%
	Warm-up	1x10, 50%
	Pyramid	1x10, 60%
	Pyramid	1x10, 70%
	Failure	1x10, 80%
	Back-off	1x20, 60%
Lying Leg Curls	Regular, finish with rest/pause	2x10, 70%
		2x8, 80% with 3 additional rest/pause reps
Machine Leg Presses	Regular	3x12-20, 70%
Romanian Deadlift	Regular	3x10-20, 60-80%
Glute Machine	Regular	2x10-12, 70-80%
Seated Machine Calf Raises	Rest/Pause	4x15-20, 60-80% with 3 additional rest/pause reps

Leg training is so demanding that it deserves a whole workout to itself. In addition, I work hamstrings, glutes, calves, and lower back with quads. That's a lot of muscle to cover. For me, there's no compelling reason to separate quads and hamstrings, although some bodybuilders do. Including lower back with legs makes sense because exercises like squats and every type of deadlift hit the whole lower back region, along with thighs and hamstrings. I contend that the deadlift is as much a leg exercise as it is a back exercise. I alternate smith machine squats with leg presses from one leg workout to the next. I occasionally do regular deadlifts in place of Romanian deadlifts. I also include a couple sets of direct glute work on the butt-blaster machine every other leg workout. Sometimes I throw in some leg extensions, but they are always light, since they tend to hurt my knees. I don't do lunges anymore, although it seems like everyone is doing them these days. Almost every time I've done them I've hurt myself, either my hamstring or knee. So, I avoid them. Besides, squats, deadlifts, and leg presses are more effective exercises overall for the quads, glutes, and hamstrings.

Workout #2, Chest & Arms		
Machine Incline Presses	Warm-up	1x10, 40%
	Warm-up	1x10, 50%
	Pyramid	1x10, 60%
	Pyramid	1x10, 70%
	Failure	1x10, 80%
	Rest/Pause	1x8, 80% with 3 additional rest/pause reps
	Back-off	1x20, 60%
Machine Bench Presses	Regular	2x12-20, 60-70%
Cable Crossovers	Regular	3x10-12, 70-80%
Alternating Dumbbell Curls (Superset with Tricep Pushdowns)	Warm-up	1x10, 60%
	Regular	2x10, 80%
Tricep Pushdown	Warm-up	1x10, 60%
	Regular	2x12-15, 70%
Barbell Curls (Superset with Dips)	Regular	1x10, 80%
	Failure	1x10, 80%
	Rest/Pause	1x8, 80% with 3 additional rest/pause reps
Dips (body weight)	Regular	3x as many reps as possible
Machine Curls (Superset with machine dips)	Failure	1x10, 80%
	Rest/Pause	1x8, 80% with 3 additional rest/pause reps
	Back-off	1x20, 60%
Machine Dips	Failure	1x10, 80%
	Rest/Pause	1x8, 80% with 3 additional rest/pause reps
	Back-off	1x20, 60%

Training chest and arms together makes good sense due to the overlap between chest and tricep exercises and my preference for training biceps and triceps in the same workout. This is my shortest workout, lasting only about 50 minutes. For most people, this is probably their longest workout and the most prioritized. Go into any gym on a Monday evening and almost every guy in the place will be doing chest and arms. Moreover, for many trainees, chest and arms are the only body parts they work at all. Many only do back and shoulders as ancillary movements and don't work their legs at all.

This workout is relatively brief for me mainly because, unlike many lifters, I don't do endless sets of chest exercises, and I superset biceps with triceps. I am usually finished with my entire workout before some guys are finished bench pressing. One of the biggest time killers I see at the gym, especially during chest workouts, is a group of guys, often more than three, participating in a bench press party of sorts. More than three lifters is too many. It just takes too long for each to lift and change weights in between. It's nearly inevitable that in a group like this, there will be as much talking as lifting. And, don't be those guys where it's hard to tell who's really lifting the weight, the lifter or the spotter.

There are a number of good chest machines out there, like Hammer Strength, for example. When I refer to a chest machine, I am referring to plate-loaded machines. I alternate these machines among chest workouts. I occasionally do Smith machine incline presses, but they tend to hurt my shoulders. I like incline dumbbell presses (with a neutral grip) from time to time, but they pose problems as well. The biggest challenge is getting heavy dumbbells into position to do the lift. Try moving two 110 dumbbells from your thighs to your shoulders on an inclined bench. It's not easy, and it invites injury. This is a good exercise, but, once you reach a high strength level, the risk of injury outweighs any further benefit from the exercise. And I feel that heaving up heavy dumbbells into position for incline or shoulder presses wastes too much energy and actually knocks at least one rep off of the amount you could have completed. Therefore, I recommend using a bar or machine for these movements.

Guys ask me about training forearms. Certainly, you could include a couple sets of wrist curls, especially immediately following a biceps exercise. However, I don't think that training forearms directly is a good use of your limited training time. I say this because most people who have good forearms seem to have them naturally. Instead of spending time working them directly, I believe you can use your time more wisely by concentrating on gripping heavy weights. That means not using straps to enhance your grip on heavy pulling exercises until you actually need them.

Workout #3, Back & Shoulders		
Barbell Bent Rows (Smith Machine) (Superset w Dumbbell side laterals)	Warm-up	1x10, 40%
	Warm-up	1x10, 50%
	Failure	2x10, 80%
Dumbbell Side Laterals	Warm-up	1x10, 40%
	Pyramid	1x10, 60%
	Pyramid	1x10, 70%
	Failure	1x10, 80%
Low-Pulley Rows (Superset w machine shoulder presses)	Regular	1x10, 70%
	Regular	1x10, 80%
	Failure	1x10, 80%
Machine Shoulder Presses	Warm-up	1x10, 40%
	Pyramid	1x10, 60%
	Pyramid	1x10, 70%
	Rest/Pause	1x8, 80% with 3 additional reps
	Back-off	1x20, 60%
Machine or cable Pulldowns (Superset w upright rows)	Warm-up	1x10, 50%
	Pyramid	1x10, 70%
	Failure	1x10, 80%
	Rest/Pause	1x8, 80% with 3 additional rest/pause reps
Upright Rows	Regular	2x10-12, 70-80%
	Failure	1x8-10, 80%
Barbell Shrugs	Regular	3x15-20, 60-70%
Machine Pullovers (superset w rear delt movement)	Regular	2x10, 80%
Rear Delt Movement	Regular	2x10, 80%

The logic behind working back and shoulders together is the high degree of overlap. Take traps, for example. Traps are hit through both back and shoulder exercises. Rear delts are another good example. Usually done with shoulders, all pulling exercises hit them as well. Many will argue that this workout is just too much for a single session, but, once again, I enhance workout efficiency by overlapping exercises and by supersetting back and shoulder exercises together. Add to this the fact that many trainees simply perform too many exercises and sets.

Similar to my other workouts, I alternate many of my exercises from one workout to the next. The only constant for back is that I try to do two rowing movements, one overhead pull-up or pull-down movement, and a pullover or stiff-arm press down movement. My favorite rowing movements are bent rows on the Smith machine (both grips), T-bar rows, one-arm dumbbell rows, low-pulley rows, and various machine rows. For shoulders I always include a machine press of some sort, both dumbbell and machine laterals, and upright rows (with barbell or dumbbell). For traps, I like heavy barbell shrugs, and I often use the trap bar, where the arms hang to the sides instead of in front of the body. The muscle magazines often tout dumbbell shrugs, but I don't think that they are very practical, especially if you are relatively strong. Dumbbells simply don't offer enough weight, unless you happen to train at a gym that has a pair of 200s lying around. Upright rows also hit the traps pretty good. An effective superset, or pre-exhaust, if you prefer, is to do a set of upright rows followed immediately by heavy shrugs. Rear delts are hit with the rear-delt machine or occasionally with dumbbells while lying face-down on an inclined bench.

You might have noticed that I haven't mentioned abs, everyone's focus. That's because I feel that ab training is way overrated – not that having visible abs is overrated, but that working them so much and so often is. People still have the misconception that you can reduce or remove fat from a certain part of the body by working the muscles of that particular part of the body. I watch people all the time routinely hit every ab machine in the gym every time they're in the gym. It's no wonder this myth simply won't die. Nearly every piece of exercise equipment peddled in T.V. ads and infomercials is focused on the abs and reducing one's midsection. "Core" is the hot buzzword right now. Everything is about training your core, whatever that means. Your abs are simply muscles. Everyone has them, and you do not need to work them any more than any other body part. Losing the bodyfat covering the abs is the only way yours will ever become visible. I work my abs once or, at most, twice a week usually after my cardio sessions on my non-lifting days. And I only do about 3 or 4 sets.

My Training Schedule

I generally train on Monday, Tuesday, Thursday and Saturday. The gym I belong to is now open 24/7 so my workout days can and do vary in response to changes in my schedule. Since I have four days for three workouts, one workout is done twice over the course of the week. Light-to-moderate cardio – walking (either on a treadmill or outside) or the elliptical – is done on my non-lifting days. I don't recommend doing cardio and resistance workouts in the same session, as cardio interferes with muscular hypertrophy. My resistance workouts are somewhat aerobic anyway, since I train at a brisk pace, perform high reps, and superset many exercises together. Here's my training schedule for any given month:

Monday	Tuesday	Wed.	Thursday	Friday	Saturday	Sunday
Legs	Chest & Arms	Light to Moderate Cardio	Back & Shoulders	Light to Moderate Cardio	Legs	Light to Moderate Cardio
Chest & Arms	Back & Shoulders	Light to Moderate Cardio	Legs	Light to Moderate Cardio	Chest & Arms	Light to Moderate Cardio
Back & Shoulders	Legs	Light to Moderate Cardio	Chest & Arms	Light to Moderate Cardio	Back & Shoulders	Light to Moderate Cardio
Legs	Chest & Arms	Light to Moderate Cardio	Back & Shoulders	Light to Moderate Cardio	Legs	Light to Moderate Cardio

Note that each workout is performed once every 5 or 6 days. Monday and Tuesday are the only consecutive workout days of the week. The only drawback to this schedule is when back & shoulders are trained the day immediately after chest & arms. Obviously, there is a lot of overlap between these two workouts. If you work your biceps hard one day, for example, only one day's rest might not be enough rest time before training back, which relies quite a bit on the biceps. Chest and triceps trained the day before shoulders presents the same problem. Light-to-moderate cardio is performed on non-lifting days. Light-to-moderate cardio, for me, consists of one or more of the following exercises performed for approximately 30 minutes: Elliptical, treadmill walking (4 or 5% incline), trail walking, including some hills. Sunday's cardio is always a trail walk of approximately 4 miles. Given the choice, I prefer walking outdoors.

I know it is common today for trainees to work only one bodypart a day and each bodypart once a week. This type of program is promoted by pro bodybuilders in glossy muscle magazines. Keep in mind that all the muscle magazines exist for only one reason: to sell nutritional supplements. And pro bodybuilders might not be the best source of training advice for the average trainee. Not because they are not knowledgeable about training; I assure you they are. Remember that elite bodybuilders have the best genetics, including recovery ability, and most take powerful performance-enhancing drugs. They can get by with a lot more training and intensity than most of us mere mortals.

I see guys following these programs and doing way too many sets. I emphasize efficiency. If you work one body part a day for an hour a day, that comes to 5 hours a week to work the entire body. With my program, I train my entire body in only 3 hours a week. And my workouts are more intense because I train at a faster pace. So, I firmly believe that by training only one bodypart at a time, you are doing too many sets and probably not working hard enough or fast enough to make significant progress.

Workout Efficiency

I can't overemphasize the importance of workout efficiency. Efficiency is an integral part of productivity, and there are several ways to make your workouts more efficient. To the most feasible extent, one should try to perform the greatest amount of work in a the shortest amount of time. To accomplish this, I strongly recommend that you employ the overlap principle as much as practical in your training. The overlap principle occurs when one exercise works more than one body part. Take deadlifts, for example. When performed correctly, deadlifts hit several major muscle groups, i.e. lats, traps, low-back, thighs, glutes, and hamstrings. This makes the exercise much more demanding and thus increases your metabolic rate and hormone response. Another good example is the dip. Are dips primarily a chest or a tricep exercise? They are both. So, you group triceps with chest and work both, equally, with one exercise. Upright rows work both shoulders and traps nearly equally. This is the essence of the overlap principle – getting two for one and thus increasing workout efficiency. Use this strategy liberally. One caveat, though, is to be careful not to combine resistance and cardio training in the same workout, since cardio tends to interfere with muscular hypertrophy. Certainly, you can do some light cardio as a warm-up prior to your regular resistance workout. If you do your cardio sessions immediately after your resistance workouts, keep the cardio fairly light and relatively brief. You are much better off to do your cardio sessions at another time of day, or better yet, on your non-lifting days.

As I outlined in my own workout, I group body parts that are related, like chest and triceps, for example. By training one body part, you naturally train the other. This decreases the number of sets you need to perform. Some advocate a push/pull routine, whereby they group chest, shoulders and tris together and back and biceps together. This does appear to be logical, but I've never liked it very much. After training chest, my shoulders are too fatigued to press my normal weight, and after training back, my biceps are too tired to do much at all.

Supersets – performing two exercises without rest – is an effective method for enhancing efficiency. I prefer to superset separate body parts, like shoulders and back or biceps and triceps. The logic is that doing a back movement doesn't impede a shoulder movement. In other words, you can follow one with the other without resting and the second exercise will not suffer. Decreasing rest time makes your workout shorter and more intense. Additionally, cutting rest time helps to build your aerobic capacity, with having to do a lot of extra (and often unnecessary) cardio. Even when not doing supersets, one should train at a reasonably fast pace.

The Most Effective Training Tactics for Gaining Muscle

While all of these tactics can be very effective at stimulating muscle growth, most serious bodybuilders, including me, prefer some over others. I've already listed the ones I use on a regular basis. So I have listed them, along with some others I use occasionally, in descending order in terms of how I rate their effectiveness.

- **Training to Failure**: This is not the most intense tactic on the list, but it represents a required threshold of intensity. On your heaviest, most intense working sets, it should be your goal to train to failure – the point where you cannot perform another rep on your own. We can debate whether more intense training tactics are even necessary, but training to failure appears to be necessary for maximizing muscular hypertrophy. Be careful, though, not to overdo it. You should train to failure on only 3-4 sets per body part trained.
- **Forced Reps**: This is the natural extension of training to failure – having someone help you eke out a couple of reps that you could not have accomplished on your own. The problem with this technique is that you need someone to assist you.
- **Partial Reps**: Like forced reps, this technique extends the set past the point of failure, this time by completing partial reps, usually in the movement's strongest position. Take the leg press as an example: You fail after completing 10 full-range reps. But instead of racking the weight, you complete a few more partial reps by only doing the upper half or third of the movement. This is a convenient and efficient way to extend sets and make your training much more demanding, not to mention, painful.
- **Rest/Pause**: This is one of my favorite training tactics, since it's perfect for those of us who train alone and who often use machines. Done at the end of a regular set, rest pauses are inserted to help you recover just long enough to do another rep, and so on until you absolutely fail. At this point forced reps could be employed to extend the set even further. Rest/pause reps can also be employed from the beginning of the set, which allows you to use more weight. I prefer a rest of approximately 3 to 5 seconds between reps, and I count it out.
- **Supersets**: I employ supersets mainly to save time – to get more work done in less time. I prefer to superset opposing body parts,

like biceps with triceps, for example, or thighs and hamstrings.

- **Descending Sets**: Also called working down the rack (when using dumbbells). Like other techniques, this involves taking a set beyond failure, this time by decreasing the weight. Take, for example, when doing curls, you fail after 8 reps with 40-pound dumbbells; you then immediately pick up the 30s and knock out another 6 to 8 reps; then pick up the 20s and go to failure.
- **Pyramid Sets**: This is one of the oldest techniques around, and for good reason; it works. Start with a light weight and higher reps on your first set and increase the weight while decreasing the reps on subsequent sets until you reach a weight where you can only get 3 or 4 reps. I don't recommend going too low on reps, as it only invites injury. After your heaviest set, you can then do a reverse pyramid. I always do at least one back-off set after my heaviest set, which usually consists of 15-20 reps done to failure. This high-rep set really leaves you with a deep muscle burn and pump. Pyramid sets and reps for squats might look something like this (after two warm-up sets): Set 1) 225 x10; 2) 275x8; 3) 315x6; 4) 335x4; 5) 225x20. The beauty of this system is that it provides for a wide rep range, which trains both fast- and slow-twitch muscle fibers and provides variety for the trainee.
- **Negative-Only Training**: Research has shown that the eccentric (negative or lowering) part of the rep produces the most damage to the muscle and thus is thought to contribute more to hypertrophy than the concentric, or positive, part of the rep. So why do the positive part of the rep at all? The positive part contributes a lot to hypertrophy as well, and negative-only training would be too demanding, not to mention impractical. The most common method to use negatives is to do a couple of negatives at the end of a set after reaching failure. This requires someone to help you move the weight during the positive portion and make sure the weight doesn't fall on you, since you are past failure at this point.

  By far, the most important thing is to accentuate the negative part of the rep during all sets. For most exercises, I advocate a 2-second positive and 2-second negative rep. Some have advocated much slower reps, like a 4-second positive and a 6-second negative. The super slow method gained some popularity by having trainees perform 10-second positive and negative reps. This goes a bit too far for me. This might be helpful for beginners who are learning proper technique. However, when you move the weight too slowly, the amount of weight and force created are decreased, and both are crucial for muscular hypertrophy.
- **Pre-Exhaust**: This technique has been around for a long time, and

almost everyone involved in weight lifting has utilized it at some point. A pre-exhaust set is actually a superset where one does an isolation exercise for a particular bodypart immediately followed by a compound, or multi-joint, exercise for the same bodypart. The idea is that the isolation exercise fatigues the target muscle almost completely, and then the compound movement, which relies on other muscles to help the target muscle, can fatigue the target muscle even more thoroughly. A common example is dumbbell flyes followed by bench presses. The pecs are fatigued by the first exercise and then further fatigued by the bench press, which involves the delts and triceps that combine to help the pecs.

In theory, pre-exhaust seems very logical. However, studies conducted using MRI technology on working muscles have shown that the degree of muscle fiber activation during a pre-exhaust set is not as impressive as when done while doing a traditional set of bench presses using 80 percent of one's 1-rep max. By limiting the amount of weight you can use during the compound lift, pre-exhaust training actually decreases your potential for hypertrophy.

- **Giant Sets/Circuit Training**: Both of these techniques involve the grouping of exercises into a circuit and performing them one after another without rest until a full circuit is completed. The difference is that with giant sets, all the exercises are for the same body part, and with circuit training, most or all of the exercises are for different body parts. Giant sets are similar to pre-exhaust training, only with more exercises, and the same limitations apply. The main reasons for doing this type of training are to get a lot of work done in a short amount of time, to burn a lot of calories, and to enhance cardiovascular fitness. Crossfit training, for example, is based primarily on this type of training.

Beginner Workout

For the beginning weight trainer, it is important to learn how to perform the lifts correctly. Therefore, I recommend starting slowly, concentrate on learning a few basic lifts, and then incorporating new lifts as those are mastered. Beginner trainees have the advantage that their muscles have not been stressed in a way that weight training does, and, therefore, in the beginning is when lifters are likely to experience their best gains. From the beginning of one's training, progress depends on continually increasing the stress applied to your muscles, as outlined in the core principles for muscle growth. This translates into another general principle: One should not do more than is necessary to stimulate muscle growth. Most beginners can make good progress by doing just a few basic exercises and few sets of each. But, how often do we see people join a gym and immediately jump into a lifting routine that would have killed Arnold Schwarzenegger. Only do what is necessary and no more. Based on this important principle, here is a basic training routine for beginners.

Exercise	Sets and Reps	Notes
Squats (barbell or Smith machine)	3x8-12	Perform two warm-up sets and pyramid up to the heaviest set of 8 reps.
Bench Press	3x8-12	Perform two warm-up sets and pyramid up to the heaviest set of 8 reps.
Deadlift	3x6-10	Perform one warm-up set and then pyramid the weight by doing 10, 8, and then 6 reps.
Bent Barbell Rows	2x8-12	Perform one warm-up set, one set of 12 and one set of 8-10.
Barbell Curls	2x8-12	Perform two sets of 8-12 reps.

The beginner workout is simple yet effective. It features compound exercises, ones that work several muscle groups at once. The five exercises work the entire body in one session. The entire workout should take only about 40 minutes to complete. One should rest about 3 minutes between sets of squats and deadlifts, by far the most demanding exercises. One should rest about 2 minutes between all sets of the other exercises. No high-intensity techniques – like forced or negative reps – are necessary at this point. This workout should be performed 3 days a week on nonconsecutive days – Monday, Wednesday, and Friday, for example. As stated before, you should focus on learning how to perform the exercises correctly. The next priority, and always a priority, is to gradually lift more weight.

You can make great gains on this program, and as you get stronger, your workouts will become more intense. To compensate for this increase in intensity, you must actually train less often in order to give your muscles enough time to recuperate and grow. At this point I recommend moving to a split routine where you train basically half your body in one workout and the other half in another workout. In this format you train four days a week – instead of three – but you train each bodypart only twice a week. I recommend upper- and lower-body workouts and incorporating new exercises and the rotation of exercises to bring variety and new stimuli to your workouts. The following is an example of a split routine, featuring two separate workouts: upper body (chest, back, shoulders, and arms) and lower body (thighs, hamstrings, lower back, glutes, calves, and abs).

Upper Body		
Exercise	**Sets and Reps**	**Notes**
Bench Press	4x8-12	Perform 2 warm-up sets and then pyramid up to your heaviest set.
Dips	2x as many as possible	Some gyms have a dip/chin assistance machine.
Pullups	2x as many as possible	Machine pulldowns may be substituted, but focus on pulling up your bodyweight.
Barbell Bent Rows	3x8-12	May be done on a Smith machine.
Shoulder Presses	3x8-12	Perform 1 warm-up set and pyramid to your heaviest set.
Upright Rows	2x8-12	May be performed with a straight bar, curl bar, or dumbbells.
Barbell Curls	4x8-12	Perform 1 warm-up set
Lying Tricep Extensions	4x8-12	Perform 1 warm-up set

Both workouts feature basic compound exercises with a few more movements thrown in to increase volume and variety.

Lower Body		
Exercise	**Sets and Reps**	**Notes**
Squats	5x6-12	Perform 2 warm-up sets then pyramid up in weight and down in reps, i.e. 12, 10, 8, 6. Then do a back-off set of 20 reps.
Deadlifts	3x6-10	Pyramid 10, 8, 6 while increasing weight.
Leg Extensions	3x10-12	70-80% of max.
Leg Curls	3x8-12	To save time these can be supersetted with calf raises.
Calf Raises	3x15-20	I believe in higher reps for calves.
Ab Crunches	2x as many as possible	Do these on a bench or in the floor and try to bring you knees back as you bring your torso forward.

During the split-training routine, you should incorporate new exercises and begin the habit of alternating exercises for the same body parts. This will help bring variety to your workouts and keep your muscles guessing as to how they will be stimulated. As presented in the following table, I recommend substituting the following secondary exercises for the primary exercises every other workout.

Primary Exercise	**Substitute Exercise**
Squat	Leg Press
Deadlift	Romanian Deadlift
Bench Press	Incline Bench Press
Barbell Bent Row	T-Bar Row, Low-Pulley Row, or One-Arm Dumbbell Row
Shoulder Press	Dumbbell Shoulder Press, Upright Row, Dumbbell Side Laterals
Barbell Curls	Dumbbell Curls
Lying Tricep Extension	Dips, Cable Pushdowns

Complete Bodyweight Workout

This workout can be done in the comfort of your living room with no additional equipment required. However, dumbbells and a chin-up bar will add to the variety of exercises, and which can also increase the intensity of your workouts. While there are a myriad of exercises that could be included, I have selected eight here simply as an example workout. The key is to move from one exercise to the next with little or no rest. Start out by performing 10 repetitions per exercise. Complete one set of each exercise without rest (1 circuit) and then rest 1 minute. Begin with one circuit and work your way up to several circuits. You should also try to increase the repetitions of each exercise. Eventually, you will gauge your progress by how many reps and circuits you complete in a prescribed period of time, say 30 minutes. To add variety, incorporate new exercises and combine this workout with other exercises like running, walking, cycling, yoga, etc.

Bodyweight Workout			
Exercise	**Rep Count**		
	Beginning	**Intermediate**	**Advanced**
Jumping Jacks	10	25	50
Push-ups	10	20	30
Mountain Climbers	10	20	30
Crunches	10	20	30
Squats	10	20	30
Alternate Toe Touches	10	20	30
Lunges	10	20	30
Standing Knee-ups	10	20	30

Common Training Mistakes

- **Not training with enough intensity**: I see this one more than any others. Most people I see in the gym seem to just be going through the motions. I rarely see people sweat, unless they've been doing an hour of cardio, which may be doing them more harm than good. Your workouts should be hard. You are trying to get your body to change, and I assure you, it doesn't want to. You have to push it, and that means doing the really difficult exercises and doing them until it burns like crazy.
- **Doing too much cardio**: Everyone needs some regular cardio for cardiovascular health and to burn more calories. However, if you are trying to build muscle – which should be everyone's primary goal – then too much cardio can compromise your gains. Many people, especially women, perform tons of cardio while doing little, if any, resistance training thinking that it is better for losing weight. Most who do this end up losing more muscle than fat, giving them the dreaded "skinny fat" look. This look is achieved when someone has lost weight and inches, but they look basically the same as they did before because they actually have less muscle than they did when they started.
- **Talking/socializing too much**: This one goes hand-in-hand with not training hard enough. You should rest some between sets, but engaging in a 20-minute conversation will not help you reach your fitness goals. Of course, some people are at the gym only to socialize, and it's a good environment for that. It's quite all right to talk to people while working out. I do. But I keep it to a minimum. You don't have to be anti-social, but always be mindful that your workout is your first priority. Socialize when your workout is over.
- **Performing the wrong exercises**: This goes further than simply emphasizing cardio over resistance training. Many people forego the more productive, harder exercises for the less productive, easier ones. You don't see a lot of people doing deadlifts, and there's never a line to use the squat rack. People seem to prefer concentration curls and ab crunches. Some ineffective exercises include the thigh adductor (bringing the legs toward each other) and the thigh abductor (pushing the legs away from each other). These exercises are targeted toward women and are a total waste of time. People wanting to develop or shape their legs and butt should be doing squats, leg presses, hamstring curls, and lunges. Many people do dozens of ab exercises (far too many), and most of them are a waste of time. People do side bends with dumbbells and twisting exercises thinking that these exercises will firm up their

love handles. To the contrary, these exercises may actually make the area larger. The only way to reduce this area is to lose the fat around the area, which means that one has to reduce caloric intake and continue to train intensely.

- **Performing goofy exercises**: I see it in the gym all the time, people doing goofy, ineffective exercises. Now, I admit that I occasionally perform unique exercises, ones that you don't see very often. I'm constantly thinking about how to use the existing equipment in the gym to come up with new, and, hopefully, more productive exercises. And often, simply doing a different exercise breaks up the monotony of your routine. There's a big difference, though, between novel and goofy. I describe goofy exercises as those that are clearly less effective (often because they are easier) than more traditional exercises, may even be dangerous, and often involve some piece of equipment that shouldn't be part of any serious gym. Some examples include these stability balls (or whatever they are called) that people lay on while doing regular exercises. The idea is that this will improve stability and increase performance in the lift. This premise is blatantly false and only enhances the risk of injury.
- **Using ludicrous form**: I'll be honest; many experienced bodybuilders use terrible form and try to tell people to use good form. I have been guilty of poor form from time to time. However, there is a big difference between using a little momentum and swing here and there and not even controlling the weight at all. I think experienced lifters learn how to cheat and still control the weight, whereas inexperienced lifters don't. A little bit of cheating, especially on the last few reps of a set, can add greatly to the intensity of the set. So, my advice to beginners is learn how to do the exercises correctly and strictly, and when you really learn how to feel the movements, you can loosen up your form a little.
- **Doing too many sets for certain bodyparts**: This seems to contradict the advice on training intensity, but it has nothing to do with intensity. Some people do far too many sets but none of them at a level of intensity high enough to do them much good. At best they're just burning calories. I see some guys in the gym doing every exercise in the book, especially on chest day. Heck, I can usually complete three bodyparts before some guys get finished with chest. Not all sets need to be done at maximum intensity, like warm-up sets, for example. However, the general principle here is that a certain threshold for intensity must be met, but it can and should be met in only a few sets for each bodypart. In general, people would be better served to do fewer sets but to work much

harder.

- **Not training legs**: It's amazing to me how many people who don't train their legs at all. You see these guys doing bench presses and curls all day while they have toothpicks for legs. Leg training involves the largest muscles in the body, so it can be brutally demanding, i.e. painful. People don't realize that by training their legs other body parts benefit simply due to the overall effect and the stimulation of growth factors like testosterone, growth hormone, and IGF-I.
- **Specializing in certain lifts at the expense of others**: As the case with avoiding leg training, many trainers focus too much attention on their chest and arms. And then most people tend to focus on their strong parts while neglecting their weak ones.
- **Overtraining**: If you train too often, and with too much intensity, you can overtrain by not allowing your muscles, or the body's systems, enough time to recover. This is a condition that thwarts progress, suppresses your immune system, and can have other damaging effects on the body. People who train very intensely are at a greater risk of overtraining. If you train intensely – as you should – you must keep your workouts relatively brief and infrequent.
- **Training too heavy**: While most people don't train intensely enough, many are bent on attempting their max bench every workout. Come-on guys, lighten up a little, give your poor spotter a break, and do some quality reps.
- **Being inconsistent**: Most people come and go at the gym. They get ultra-motivated around New Year, join a gym, workout hard for a few weeks, and then fizzle out. Some people train in cycles. They train for a couple of months – long enough to see some results – and then like clockwork they disappear. After a couple of months, they come back only to start over again. To get results, you have to train hard enough and long enough. To maintain results for the long-term, you must make fitness a priority for the rest of your life.
- **Not paying enough attention to nutrition**: Good nutrition is a must if you want to maximize your fitness potential. Proper nutrition fuels intense workouts and helps you recover and build. Whether you are trying to lose, gain, or maintain weight, you need a strategy. You must develop sound nutrition habits to go along with regular exercise.

Perspective

If you interview ten bodybuilders, you will likely get ten different training regimens. You'll see differences in exercises used, the grouping of bodyparts, number of sets performed, rep ranges, intensity-enhancing techniques, and amount of rest between sets. This variability tells me that there probably isn't a one, single best training regimen that can be prescribed for everyone to follow. On the contrary, there appears to be a multitude of training regimens that will produce results. However, if you look closely enough at those ten bodybuilders, you'll also find many commonalities in how they train and eat. It's those commonalities that I pay attention to and so should you, because that is where we unlock the secrets to muscle growth.

7. Training Myths

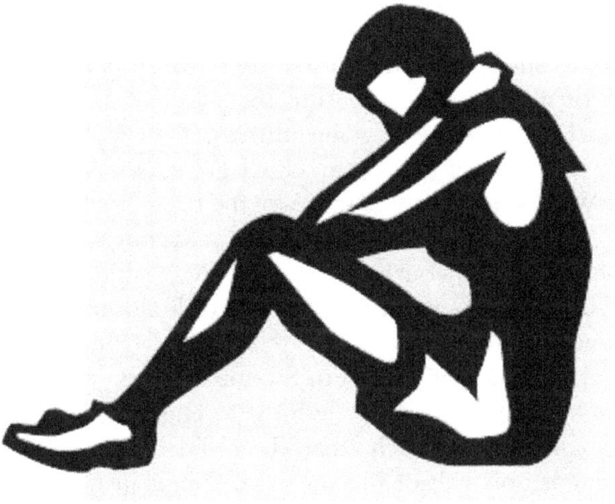

The only exercise some people get is jumping to conclusions, running down their friends, side-stepping responsibility, and pushing their luck!
– Author Unknown

Training myths and misinformation just won't die. They get passed along from one generation to the next by parents, coaches, trainers, and other well-intentioned individuals. Wiley marketers, too, in their attempt to peddle their wares to largely uninformed consumers, help to keep training myths alive by encouraging peoples' false beliefs about exercise. Here are some of the more common training myths that seemingly will not die.

- **Spot reduction is possible**: In other words, it's possible to lose fat from a specific area of the body simply by exercising that particular bodypart. Because so many people still believe this myth, unscrupulous marketers have sold millions of ab-training gadgets. Of course, no one ever reads the fine print, which states that results depend upon one's diet. Even in the gym I see people doing every ab machine in the place. Many people train their abs every workout. We all have six-pack abs, but for most people, they are buried beneath a layer of fat. The only way to ever have visible abs is to lose the fat that covers them. When you train your abs, you are burning only a few calories. So, you'd actually be better off doing exercises that burn more calories while training your abs a lot less often. When you lose fat, you lose it all over your body, not just in one particular area.

- **To get toned, you should use light weights and do high reps**: First of all, I'm not even sure that "toned" is an actual physical state of the body, or of your muscles. Your muscles, based on the demands you place on them, either grow, shrink, or maintain their size. What I think people mean by the term "toned" is the look one gets when they build some muscle through exercise, and the muscles simultaneously become more visible due to a loss of bodyfat. The most efficient way to build muscle is by using relatively heavy weights (70 to 80% of your 1-rep max) and moderate reps (8-12 per set). So, the best way to achieve the type of look that many people desire is to engage predominantly in the bodybuilding approach that I outlined previously. However, training is only half of the equation. Diet is just as important, since you must drop bodyfat in order to make your muscles more visible and give you the aesthetic look that is so in vogue.

- **Strength training will bulk women up**: This might be the most persistent myth in the fitness arena. I'd like to have a dollar for every time a women has said, "Oh, I don't want to lift weights. I don't want big muscles," I'd be a very rich man. It's unfortunate because it keeps women from reaching their physical potential and from attaining the type of body that they so desire. Heck, most men can't build big muscles, and they have a big hormonal advantage. Most women simply don't produce enough testosterone to build big muscles. What bulks women up is gaining too much fat. Women should do some cardio exercise to burn calories and enhance overall conditioning, but strength training is the only thing that will help reshape the body. You can't get this type of look by doing aerobics classes alone; only intense resistance exercise can accomplish this. In fact, women should train just like men do. By avoiding strength training, women are depriving themselves of the most productive way to achieve the type of body they want.

- **You can't gain muscle past the age of 40**: It does get a bit more difficult the older you get, but plenty of research shows that even individuals in their 70s gain muscle while on a resistance training program. The main problem for men is that their testosterone and growth hormone levels drop gradually as they age, and these hormones are very important in the muscle-building process. The good news is that hormone replacement therapy is becoming more common for men, the way it has been for women for a long time.

- **The more you sweat, the better your workout**: This one is somewhat true, although very misleading. Sweating is the primary means to cool the body. The harder you work, the more apt you are to sweat. You need to train hard, but a couple of factors influence how much you will sweat. First, some people just sweat more than others. Sweating is controlled by the sympathetic nervous system, and this varies greatly among individuals. Secondly, the higher the humidity, the more you will sweat. Think about the sultry days of summer when you sweat just getting in and out of your car. They say that sweating is healthy. If this is true, I should live forever.

- **Cardio should be done first thing in the morning on an empty stomach**: The idea behind this trend was that doing cardio while in a fasted state, you would burn more fat, since your blood glycogen levels would be low. This fasted-state condition would cause your body to burn more fat since carbohydrates would be in short supply. Recent research, though, has debunked this idea. In fact, doing cardio while in a fasted state increases the risk that you will burn hard-earned muscle. Apparently, if carbs are too low – as in a fasted state – your body starts converting amino acids into energy as much as it uses fat for energy. This is the absolute last thing you want to happen. You must do all you can to preserve your hard-earned muscle. At the end of the day, the only thing that seems to matter in regard to fat loss is whether or not you created a caloric deficit.

- **For effective fat burning you should keep your heart rate in the fat-burning zone**: Almost every piece of cardio equipment monitors your heart rate and lets you know whether you are in the fat-burning zone. For a long time now fitness experts have preached the necessity of training at 60-70 percent of your maximum heart rate for at least 20 minutes at a time. While it's true that you burn a higher percentage of fat calories while doing this, you could burn more total calories by training more intensely. This is the logic behind the now popular high-intensity interval training

(HIIT). This type of training consists of brief bursts of energy followed by periods of lower intensity movement repeated over a period of time. Remember that the only requirement for fat loss is creating a caloric deficit over time.

- **Stretching before working out is crucial to preventing injury**: This one is so ingrained in physical culture that almost everyone who exercises stretches beforehand. As it turns out, recent research shows that stretching before exercise actually reduces strength in the muscles stretched and actually increases the likelihood of injury. The best way to warm up is to perform the exercise you intend to do only at a slower pace and lighter resistance and then gradually work your way up to your desired training load. Save stretching for when your workout is over.

- **Strength is closely correlated with muscle size**: Stated another way, muscle mass increases in proportion to increases in strength. This is true but only to a degree and varies greatly among individuals. As a general rule, you should try to increase strength, since the strength of a muscle is the prime predictor of the muscle's size. Increasing the resistance is still the best way to overload a muscle. Plus, seeing your training weights increase is a great motivator, as it shows that you are making progress. All this said, though, there are many people who are very strong but don't possess muscle mass in proportion to their strength. The reverse is also true. There are many heavily-muscled lifters who aren't as strong as they look and don't use very heavy weights when training. In regard to muscular hypertrophy, strength is important, but it is only one of several important factors involved in the hypertrophy process. Other important factors include time under tension, concentrating on the negative, rest time between sets, and other factors discussed in Chapter 4.

- **Doing squats will make your butt big**: Isn't having a big butt a good thing? Let me qualify that by saying that a big, muscular butt is good, whereas a big, fat butt is bad. Along with legs, squats build the glutes (your butt), which doesn't give you the big, fat butt, rather the firm, sexy butt.

- **Muscle soreness is the best indicator of how effective your workout was**: Muscle soreness is caused by slight tears to individual muscle fibers due to intense muscular contractions. Muscle soreness indicates that damage was done, but it doesn't necessarily mean that that particular workout will lead to growth. Your body first has to repair that damage, and that process has more to do with nutrition and rest. We all know that we get sore when we first begin an exercise program or even do a different exercise. The longer we train, the more our muscles become resistant to soreness. However, that doesn't mean that my workouts are any less effective now than they were ten years ago.

- **Swimming is a great weight-loss activity**: Swimming is an excellent form of exercise and is especially well-suited for overweight individuals who have trouble walking or doing other movements where they must support their entire bodyweight. The buoyancy of water partly supports one's body weight and thus eases the pressure on joints. This benefit does have one drawback for those trying to lose weight. Because the water supports part of your bodyweight, you end up burning fewer calories while in the water than you would exercising out of water. So, if you are trying to lose weight and you like to swim, go ahead and hit the pool but also include other forms of exercise where you have to support your entire bodyweight.

- **A cardio workout boosts your metabolism for hours after completing the workout**: This has been touted for a long time but has been highly exaggerated. It's true that cardio exercise does rev up your metabolism to an extent. Your body heats up, you perspire, and it takes a while for your body to cool down and return to normal. Of course, the amount of time this takes depends on the intensity and duration of your workout. In truth, resistance exercise has a much greater potential to boost metabolism for a greater period of time. After an intense resistance workout your body goes into action to heal the damage that was done to the muscles during the workout. This process involves a myriad of chemical processes occurring throughout the body, and which takes a while to complete. Also, any additional muscle helps to boost your metabolism because it requires additional calories, nutrients, and various chemicals and chemical processes in order to maintain it. Having more muscle really does burn more calories, even while resting.

Perspective

Everything I've presented in this chapter can be supported by research. However, I realize that gym lore is resilient, especially when it gets repeated often enough. This is why it is so important for you think critically about fitness. You must ask the right questions and stay up to date on current research. Read, read, read, but be cognizant of the sources.

8. ONGOING DEBATES

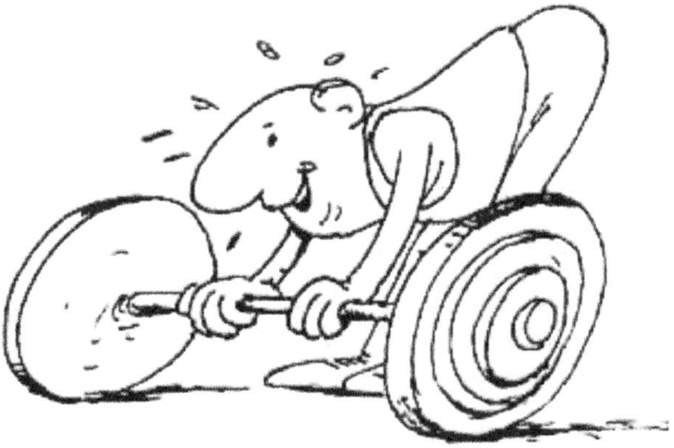

Free Weights versus Machines

Just to clarify, a free weight is a barbell, a dumbbell, a kettlebell, or your own bodyweight. Everything else is a machine. I've heard most of my life that free weights are more effective than machines at building muscle. Some research leans in this direction, but, even if this is true, I don't know if it trumps the benefits offered by machines. In my view, here are the advantages of machines over free weights:

- **Saves time**: You don't have to change weight plates, and even if you use plate-loaded machines, it's generally much easier and faster to get plates on and off. Reducing the time between sets makes your workout shorter and potentially more intense.
- **Safer**: Those who advocate free weights claim that they are safer than machines. I don't see it this way. When lifting free weights, one must learn to balance the weight as it moves through the range of motion. In my experience, most injuries occur while lifting free weights when the weight momentarily becomes unbalanced, deviates from its normal trajectory, and thus places undue stress on a stabilizer muscle, or, commonly, connective tissue, like a tendon. With machines, balance is not an issue. I haven't done heavy bench presses in years due to severe shoulder pain. However, I can do

heavy machine chest exercises – like Hammer Strength, for example – because the pain I feel while doing the free weight version is exacerbated by me having to balance the weight.

- **Focuses on the target muscle**: The balance issue comes into play again. With machines, you can focus all your attention on working the muscle. Even a novice lifter can perform machine exercises with good form. The same can't be said for free weights, as one must "learn" how to perform the exercise correctly. Some claim that the balancing act muscles perform while lifting free weights contributes to muscle growth, but I think that this effect is overrated. Muscles respond to stimuli applied to them. Muscles can't determine from where the stimuli originate, free weights or machines. So, the key is to place muscles under the greatest stress, while minimizing the risk of injury. I firmly believe that machines can produce similar degrees of stress as compared to free weights, and they can do it more safely and timely.

Gym Versus Home Training

While you can get fit without joining a gym, I believe that a commercial gym offers several important advantages to working out at home. And let me state that when I refer to a "commercial" gym, I am referring to well-run fitness facility that has a wide variety of equipment and an atmosphere conducive to training and health promotion. Obviously, not all gyms meet these criteria. So, when looking for a gym to train at, look for one that has a clean environment, has a wide array of equipment (including cardio pieces), has equipment that is well maintained, and has personal trainers available, if needed. A good gym has the following advantages:

- Variety of equipment, including free weights, weight machines, and cardio equipment. I can't stress how important this is. I've tried training at home, but I get bored very quickly due to the lack of equipment.
- A good training environment: A well-run gym is clean, has ample space, and other people training. I enjoy training around others. You can derive motivation by training around others. There's a certain camaraderie shared by trainees. Trainees support each other.
- A gym is a good learning environment. Most gyms have personal trainers for individualized instruction and classes. Training with others gives you the opportunity to watch what others do and to ask questions. Just be careful who you ask for training advice.

- A gym membership is relatively inexpensive, especially when you consider how much money you can shell out for home exercise equipment. For about a dollar a day you can have access to a wide range of commercial-grade equipment. Another problem with home exercise equipment is that much of it is of low quality. I think that most of the companies that specialize in home exercise equipment don't expect consumers to actually utilize their products on a regular basis. Most of this stuff ends up as a clothes hanger in someone's bedroom.

I can't imagine not training at a gym. The gym is an environment where I feel right at home. Even when I'm traveling, I get in a workout at a local gym. I like to use different pieces of equipment than I'm used to and wish that my home gym had certain pieces that I like. I can't emphasize enough the importance of having a wide variety of equipment. For many, half the struggle of working out is beating boredom. To reach your physical potential, you need all of the training tools that a good gym provides.

Training Partner Versus Going Solo

I must admit that I like training alone. By "alone" I mean without a training partner. I enjoy training around other people, and I love the atmosphere of gyms. Over the years I have had many training partners, some lasting longer than others. I've actually had guys train a few times with me or until we did an exceptionally brutal leg workout, and then they weren't so eager to train with me.

I don't have anything against people having a training partner. Training partners support and encourage each other and spot one another during heavy lifts. While I acknowledge these benefits, I'd like to make an argument for training alone. With regard to my training, it's all up to me. Whether I make progress or not is up to me and me alone. I like that feeling – the feeling that I am completely responsible for my own progress. I don't have to depend on anyone for anything. I don't have to wait on my partner to arrive at the gym before I begin training. In fact, I can train anytime I want. I love that flexibility. If I want to alter my program, I don't have to explain my reasoning to anyone. If I need a spot (and that isn't all that often), I simply ask someone.

No matter what I say, I realize that many trainees will want to train with a partner, and that's all right with me. For those who do, here's what I recommend: Train with someone who has similar goals and the same training philosophy. That way, both of you will be on the same page. Refrain from group training. The old saying "two's company and three's a crowd" is true in regard to working out, too. When you get too many training together, inevitably there is too much talking, too much resting, and not enough lifting. The workout becomes more of a social gathering, more like a round of golf with the guys than an intense workout. And there's no need to spot your partner on every set. Let him or her do the work and provide slight assistance only on the most demanding sets, and that should only be a few sets each workout. Above all, don't lift the weight for your partner. Sometimes it's hard to tell who's doing the most work, the lifter or the spotter. I've witnessed many times guys performing the bench press and the spotter essentially doing a deadlift trying to get the bar up far enough to rack it.

Do You Need a Personal Trainer?

When I owned my gym, I trained people more on an informal basis than on a client-trainer basis. My primary goal was to demonstrate how to train properly and safely so gym members could get the most out of their workouts. At the gym where I currently train I still get a lot of questions about training and nutrition. As much as I enjoy helping others with their training, I don't think that I would want to do it full-time. Personal trainers provide a valuable service in teaching and encouraging their clients. However, I also believe that people can become too dependent on a trainer, in that they can't train without one. In just a few sessions, a good trainer can show someone how to do a wide variety of exercises and set them up with a good training routine. There's no need to keep a trainer indefinitely. At some point you have to take off the training wheels and go on your own.

Training Journal

As a way to keep track of progress, many trainees keep very detailed records of each workout, including the specific exercises, weights used for each set, and the total time for the workout. This way, you always know how much weight you used and how much you should shoot for in your next workout. Journal entries can also describe how you felt during the workout, i.e. did the weights feel heavy or light. It's also common for trainees to document what and how much they eat and how they feel and look based on the particular foods they eat or supplements they take.

Obviously, a training journal can be beneficial, but it does take discipline to keep up with it and make entries during your workout. It also takes time from your workout. I've tried to keep a journal from time to time, but I always had trouble keeping up with it, and I never felt that it helped my progression very much. If you look around the gym, you'll see that the majority of trainees don't keep a journal. So, I don't think that a journal is necessary, by any means, for you to make progress. However, if it helps to motivate you, then I encourage you to keep one. I have an example of a training log in Chapter 13.

Periodization

Periodization has become a common phrase in discussions involving training and cuts across athletics and all sorts of fitness programs. The general idea of periodization is that one's training should be divided into distinct periods of time where one changes his or her training protocols in order to expose the body to different training stimuli. These periods, often called cycles, can last anywhere from a few weeks to a few months. Most competitive athletes, for example, alter their training from pre-season to in-season to off-season. It is thought that by periodically and systematically varying training stimuli, trainees can keep the body guessing and force it to adapt to changing demands. These changes in training can amount to changes in one or more of the following variables: training frequency, exercises, sets, reps, intensity, rest, or type of training, like more or less cardio, for example. Changes in diet may also be a consideration.

I think that periodization is overrated for just about everyone except for possibly competitive athletes. You can understand why athletes need to train differently during their competitive season than they do during the off-season. The training intensity and time necessary to make improvements in the off-season cannot be maintained during the competitive season and would actually hinder performance during competition. For non-athletes, though, those of us trying to maximize our physical potential and who are not encumbered by athletic competition, periodization does not make much sense. I base this contention on the following logic: If there is a best way to train for optimal results – in the way of exercises, sets, reps, etc. – then why would you deviate from those training protocols? Anything less will not be as productive and could very well be a waste of time. Periodization advocates might argue that different training protocols produce different results and that one cannot possibly hit all of these training varieties in single workouts. I argue that if we know the training protocols that produce the greatest gains in muscle (and we do), we should make them the basis of all workouts. If higher reps exert a desirable effect on muscular hypertrophy, then higher reps should be employed in every workout. Why wouldn't they be? The same can be said for low-to-medium reps. In other words, you must do everything you can and use every piece of knowledge you have to make your training as productive and efficient as possible.

Now that I've argued against periodization, I will admit that some people may need to vary their training more drastically in order to stave off monotony. If you feel that you are getting really bored or burned out with your current training regimen, you might consider trying a crossfit training routine for three or four weeks as a major change of pace. This will serve as a new challenge for you. You could also try a powerlifting approach for a few weeks out of the year, especially if you want to boost your strength levels. No matter if you try periodization or not, I do recommend that you take a week off from training about every four months. This periodic downtime will help your body to heal, including your nervous system. Being off for a while will also serve to reignite your motivation.

Rep Ranges

People have argued for various rep ranges, but most of the information out there is based on anecdotal experience. Fortunately, science has looked at this question extensively, and the answer lies somewhere between the two extremes. As it turns out, low reps (1-5) are best for building strength, with powerlifters serving as good examples. High reps (13+) are best for building endurance. Mid-range reps (6-12) are best for enhancing muscular hypertrophy, as the way most bodybuilders train.

So, the answer to the question depends primarily on your goals. Do you want to gain mainly strength, endurance, or muscle? My personal preference is to train mainly in the mid-range, but sometimes I do lower reps, and I often do higher reps. Therefore, my prioritization is first mid-range, then higher reps, and, finally, lower reps.

Much of this discussion about rep ranges depends on the amount of weight used. Obviously, the more reps you do, based on your max, the less weight you can handle. Weight is just one variable in this discussion. Another important variable is time under tension, or the amount of time the muscle is under stress for a particular set. In the end, the number of reps performed doesn't really matter as much as the amount of time the muscle is under direct tension. If you do your reps slower, for example, especially the negative part of the lift, that increases the amount of time under tension, regardless of the number of reps performed.

Turn Down the Volume

Traditionally, bodybuilders have done a high number of sets in their workouts, but there is a trend now to do fewer sets but train more intensely. Called high-intensity training (HIT), trainees often do no more than one set per bodypart, after two or more warm-up or pyramid sets. This one working set is typically taken at least to failure and often beyond, with forced reps, rest/pause reps, and/or negatives. This practice can work, and many trainees like it. However, I still believe that those interested primarily in muscular hypertrophy should do more sets. I like the idea of one all-out working set per exercise, but some people get carried away. There's no need to take every set to failure. In fact, doing so is ultimately counterproductive as it inevitably leads to overtraining. You need more variety in your workouts than HIT provides. Some sets need to be higher reps, some mid-range, and a few lower reps. The reps are what builds muscle, and you need a high number of reps per bodypart, and this demands more than only one working set per bodypart.

Tighten Your Belt

You need a lifting belt, but you don't need to wear it as often as you think. The purpose of wearing a belt is to tighten the muscles around your core and thus support your lower back and abs. Therefore, the belt is needed only when the low back is in jeopardy, like when doing exercises where you have to bend at the waist, squat, or lift a heavy object overhead while standing. I always wear a belt when doing squats, deadlifts, bent rows, overhead presses, and shrugs.

Just because I recommend wearing a belt while doing certain exercises, doesn't mean that you have to do the same. Many people never wear a belt.

1. Wearing a belt will help decrease the risk of injury to the lower back.
2. Wearing a belt will enable you to lift more weight in the exercises I mentioned above.
3. Wearing a belt will give you the confidence to attempt heavier weights.

Some people get carried away and wear a belt for all of their sets. This is completely unnecessary and can even be non-productive. If you wear a belt for all or most of your sets, you never allow the muscles of the core to fully develop. You probably don't realize it, but your abs are working during many of the exercises you do for other bodyparts.

Gym Etiquette

Over the years I've seen about every kind of personality and behavior in the gym. Most people who work out in a gym are courteous and accommodating. There's always a few, though, who exhibit unacceptable behaviors. It's often the bad behaviors of a very few that discourage many more people from working out at a gym. While we all have our pet peeves, here is a list of common do's and don'ts at the gym:

- **Rack your weights**: Not racking your weights might be the biggest offense in the gym, and one, unfortunately, that is still too common. Don't you just love the guy who loads up the leg press with 20 45-pound plates and doesn't take them off when he finishes? It's a complete workout for the next person just to unload it. And many women have trouble lifting and moving 45-pound plates. There's nothing more inconsiderate to other lifters in the gym than to leave your weights on the equipment. The only exception to this rule is when someone asks who to leave a certain amount of weight on the equipment for them to use. In this case, you are helping them, since they don't have to load the equipment with the desired weight. They now, however, assume responsibility for unloading the weight.

- **Noise**: Some people, mainly guys, make too much noise in the gym. This usually consists of over-exaggerated grunting or screaming while lifting. It could also be the excessive clanging of weights or abruptly dropping them. When guys are exerting maximum effort, a little grunting is expected and completely permissible. What I object to are these guys who have to draw attention to themselves by making loud, Neanderthal noises. No one wants to hear this, and it gives bodybuilders and powerlifters a bad name. By all means, train hard and heavy, but practice some self-discipline in respect to noise.
- **Socializing**: The gym can be an ideal place to interact with friends and to meet new people. Some of my closest friendships started and were cultivated at the gym. The problem comes when the only reason you go to the gym is to socialize. You've no doubt seen these people. They do a lot of talking and very little, if any, training. What's worse, their constant jabbering keeps others from training as well. I've actually had some of these jokers accost me right in the middle of a heavy set. Talk about breaking someone's focus. There's nothing wrong with being friendly and talking with others between sets, but it should be kept to minimum.
- **Working-In**: This is the term for when someone wants to do a set on the piece of equipment you are using while you are resting between sets. It is considered good etiquette for you to allow someone to work in, but they should ask if it's okay. Keep in mind, though, that when you work in with someone, you shouldn't expect them to change the weight very much, as in adding or taking off plates. This takes time, and the person might be trying to keep a brisk pace. This isn't a problem on weight-stack machines where all it takes to change the weight is simply pulling a pin. It's also considered good etiquette to ask another lifter if they are still using a piece of equipment before you begin using it. It's okay to ask

someone on a piece of equipment how many sets they have left. They will either tell you how many or invite you to work in. What's aggravating is when someone camps out on a piece of equipment doing set after set and not budging in between sets. This is considered very poor etiquette: The equipment hogs. When using a piece of equipment, especially a weight-stack machine, you should always get off the machine between sets. This way, others feel welcome to work in.

- **Spotting**: It is generally good etiquette to spot someone when asked. One caveat here would be your level of experience in knowing how to spot someone on the particular lift that they are attempting. Spotting can be tricky, depending on the lift and the lifter. It is perfectly acceptable to tell someone asking for a spot that you don't feel confident that you can ensure the safety of the lifter. When I ask someone for a spot, which isn't very often, it's always someone I know and someone who I know can do what I want. Often, as in the bench press, a spot simply involves the spotter providing a bare minimum of help with the lift. Some lifters expect too much help from their spotters, and the spotter ends up, essentially, performing the last two reps and racking the bar. In these cases, the strength of the spotter becomes paramount. Other lifts, like the squat, for example, are especially dangerous. One must lift the weight, walk away from the supports, perform a certain number of reps, and then walk forward and rack the weight. In these cases, you want a spotter who has done this before. As a final note on spotting, before asking someone to spot you, be courteous and sensitive to their workout. Ask them when they are between sets, and don't wear them out. There have been times when I've spotted guys bench pressing for 5 or more sets. That's too much; you have to allow people to get their own workout in without undue interference.
- **Sweating**: I know that I griped before about people not sweating enough, but have you ever wanted to use a piece of equipment in the gym only to find it drenched in sweat from the schmuck who just used it and didn't wipe it off? If you leave sweat on a piece of equipment, please wipe it off when finished. The gym should have paper towels and disinfectant to wipe off the equipment after use. If not, carry a towel with you.
- A related question is whether people should wipe down the equipment with disinfectant after each use, even if they didn't sweat on it. After all, germs are spread primarily through hand contact, which puts more emphasis on cleaning hand grips. If the gym provides disinfectant, in the form of spray or wipes, I think it

is considered good etiquette to wipe down equipment after you are finished. This is a case where it is better to err on the side of caution. On the flip side, I don't think it is necessary for germ freaks to carry a can of disinfectant around with them spraying everything they come into contact with.

- **Clothing**: The style and amount of clothing worn in the gym varies greatly across the spectrum. The most common rule is for shirts and shoes to be worn. I've always been more concerned with comfort and utility than with fashion. Some gyms frown on women showing their midriff. Some guys are hard to figure out, like the ones who never wear shorts, even in hot weather.
- **Chalk**: The chalk used by lifters is the same stuff you see gymnasts use before they get on the bars. It improves your grip by absorbing moisture on the hands. Most serious powerlifters and bodybuilders cannot train without it. The problem is that chalk is very messy. It's hard to use without it getting all over the floor and everything else. For this reason, most gyms, except for the hardcore ones, discourage its use. I can't blame gyms for this, as a lot of chalk users aren't very responsible with it. If you are intent on using it, and I do occasionally, I recommend keeping your own stash in a small plastic container in your gym bag. Only use it on the sets when your grip is paramount and only get out enough to cover your hands. **Tip**: Chalk comes in blocks. It's less messy if you try to keep the blocks intact by rubbing the block on your hands and not breaking it up into a powder.

Perspective

Because these are debates, and they have been going on for a long time, they are likely to remain contentious well into the future. And with every debate, there are at least two sides. I have presented rationales for my personal preferences, based on my years of training. But they are just that – my personal preferences – and not necessarily yours. In the end, you must do what you think is best, no matter what I, or anyone else, says.

9. FITNESS FADS

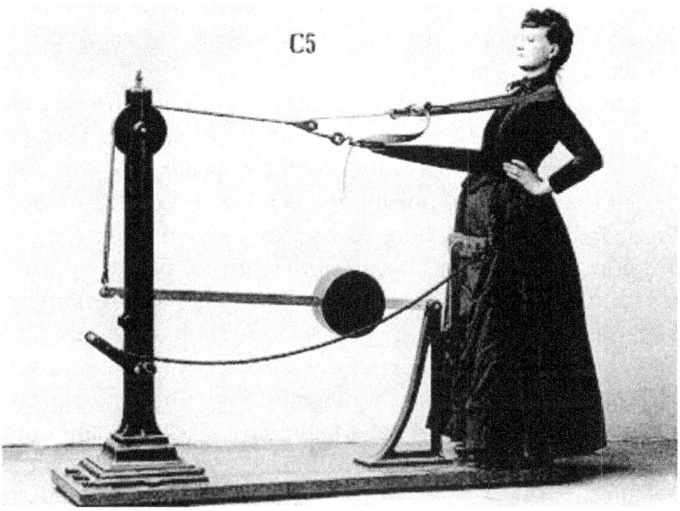

Those who think they have not time for bodily exercise will sooner or later have to find time for illness – Edward Stanley

A fad is typically defined as a fleeting fancy, something that catches on with the general public and eventually falls out of favor only to be replaced by a new fad. That's not to say that all fitness fads are worthless. On the contrary, some have been relatively effective. The thing about all fads, though, is that they suffer from a fatal flaw. They are generally hyped so highly that they can't possibly deliver the results that they promise. Some of the more effective fads are often too intense for the average trainee, and thus cannot be sustained over time.

The fitness arena has seen more than its fair share of fads, all promising to deliver results to those willing to pay for them. A myriad of exercise programs, equipment, and diets have been marketed, tweaked, and remarketed over the years. It seems as though people will buy anything, especially if it promises to make them look or feel better. All it takes is a slick infomercial with some sexy models jumping around, and people will buy it. Come up with an exercise routine, regardless of what it is – calisthenics, dance moves, kick boxing, you name it – give it a cool name, market it, and people will try it. Remember these: Jazzercise, Step Aerobics, Boot Camp, Tae Bo, Spinning, and now Zumba. Many of these group-oriented programs take on a cult-like status during their rise in popularity, or until the next best program comes along. Think about the mass following Pilates and Yoga has commanded over their lifespans. They've been around long enough that they could arguably be called philosophies as much as exercise programs.

The fitness movement in this country could rightly be called the fad fitness movement. People are desperate to find some new diet, pill, exercise regimen, or contraption that will bring them results, and this desperation is reflected in the billions of dollars we spend on every new, or recycled, diet or exercise fad that comes along and promises to make us slim and shapely. When it comes to making choices about fitness, people appear to lose all ability to think critically. How else can you explain why seemingly intelligent people repeatedly throw their money away on crazy diets, ineffective exercise equipment, and unrealistic workouts? This is exactly why I emphasize critical thinking as an integral part of any fitness plan. You have to be able to wade through the marketing hype, ask the right questions, and know where to get reliable information in order to make good decisions about fitness.

The Biggest Fitness Fads of All Time

Several media outlets have posted lists of popular fitness fads that have come and gone over the years. While "fad" carries somewhat of a negative connotation, not all these fads were bad or ineffective at promoting fitness. As I've said before, all forms of exercise can be beneficial. However, some of these fads were more effective than others, but likely none lived up to the incredible hype that they generated.

- **Aerobics**: The term was coined in 1968 by Dr. Kenneth Cooper and became the general term that describes a type of exercise – like running – that makes us breathe and conditions the heart and cardiovascular system. Cooper's work, originally directed towards astronauts, was the progenitor of the aerobics class, spurred the jogging craze of the 70's, and spawned other forms of aerobic exercise, like step, dance, and water aerobics, all of which are still popular today.
- **Jazzercise**: Founded in 1969 by Judi Sheppard Missett, Jazzercise combines elements of jazz with common aerobics. Jazzercise has had an incredibly long run but now has splintered off into other classes, like step aerobics, for example.
- **Sweatin to the Oldies**: Popularized by Richard Simmons in the

80's, this method is a lower-intensity aerobics put to older music. Simmons' name became synonymous with the aerobics-type dance class, even though he himself was always pudgy. It was his personality and enthusiasm that appealed to people.

- **Tae Bo**: Created by Billy Blanks in 1976, Tae Bo combines elements of dance, martial arts, and boxing. Variations of this type, like mixed martial arts (MMA), for example, have become popular as well. Even the hugely popular P90X and Insanity incorporate elements of kickboxing into their programs.
- **8-Minute Abs**: Supposedly, an ab workout that will help you shed inches from your waistline and reveal a defined six-pack. Don't forget the diet. Here's a tip: You don't need to pay for a special ab workout. There are no secrets out there to training your abs, or any other bodypart, for that matter.
- **Boot Camps**: These training sessions simulate military-type inductee training, commonly called "boot camp." Exercises include a lot of running, calisthenics, pushups, and plyometics, including a drill sergeant yelling at you. I guess people want to experience being in the military, but only for a few hours a week.
- **Pilates**: Created by Joseph Pilates in Germany in the early 1900's, exercises are designed to build strength and endurance and increase flexibility.
- **Spinning**: Group cycling on stationary bikes led by an instructor who motivates individuals to put forth their maximum effort. You can certainly burn a lot of calories if you don't mind being tortured. Spinning can be grueling, so participants get a sense of accomplishment after completing a workout. Personally, I never liked riding a bicycle that much. I think it's those funky, uncomfortable seats.
- **Pole Dancing Classes**: This activity, which actually mirrors the moves used by strippers, has popped up in gyms across the country. This might say more about the popularity and acceptance of stripping as a profession. There are plenty of blooper videos of women doing this at home, usually with a comical end. Part of its allure is due to women wanting to explore their sexuality, not to mention the fact that their husbands and boyfriends are encouraging them, too. In defense of pole dancing, it can be a very strenuous workout, one that enhances strength, flexibility, balance, and agility.
- **Zumba**: Created by Alberto "Beto" Perez in the 1990's, it combines elements of typical aerobics classes with Columbian dance moves. Zumba, like all other aerobics type classes, can burn

a lot of calories in a typical one-hour session. The newness of it, combined with sexy marketing, has made Zumba one of the biggest fads to come along.

- **Wii Fit**: A video game created by Nintendo where participants engage in strength training, yoga, aerobics, and balance games. The intent is to make exercise fun yet challenging and to get families to exercise together. I like to call this "virtual" fitness.
- **Yoga**: I hesitated to put yoga on the list, since it has been around virtually forever and is as much a philosophy as anything else. I put it on the list because it became very trendy in the western world in the 80's. Yoga, as practiced in exercise classes, concentrates on participants' breathing, stretching, and meditation. Yoga has been found to be beneficial in the treatment of high blood pressure, low-back pain, depression, and stress. So it's not been the worst of fads.

Dubious Fitness Equipment

- **Bow Flex**: Build muscle via flexible bands? It does provide resistance but at nowhere near the intensity of free weights or other weight machines. The commercials were very slick and persuasive, but I doubt seriously if the buffed up models got their bodies solely from using bow flex. One thing that hurts the credibility of bow flex is that the company started pushing a set of adjustable dumbbells to supplement the bow flex apparatus. Well, if the bow flex is supposed to work so well on its own, what is the need for the dumbbells? In my opinion, you would do better by purchasing and using the dumbbells alone.
- **Thigh Master**: Popularized by Suzanne Sommers, you put this gadget between your thighs and squeeze your legs together. Total waste of money and time.
- **Ab Roller**: This apparatus keeps the makes the traditional ab crunch movement very strict because of the way it "rolls" and guides the movement. You still see these things at most gyms, and I have to say that it makes the crunch movement feel like it's really targeting the abs. Although this is one of the better fads to come around, I still wouldn't think of buying it. You can work your abs very well without it, or any other piece of equipment.
- **Shake Weight**: The shake weight is a dumbbell that you shake, and it's the shaking motion that works your muscles, not the actual weight of the dumbbell providing resistance. What can I say about the Shake Weight? It has become the laughing stock of the fitness community. Even late night comics poke fun at it. There's

absolutely no science to it, but that hasn't kept it from selling.

- **Nordic Track**: Here I'm talking about the cross-country ski simulators first made famous by Nordic Track. These became extremely popular back in the 90s, as it seemed everyone had one. There was some science behind these, as cross-country skiing burns the most calories of any type of exercise. However, the machines were awkward and hard to use. I remember that it took me a while to learn the movement of pulling on the ropes with my arms while alternating my leg movements to make a fluid motion. And the thing never really caught on in gyms. Now you rarely see one. Nordic Track continues to make treadmills and other exercise equipment.
- **Total Gym**: Chuck Norris has endorsed this thing forever, and I'm not one who wants to anger Chuck Norris. This thing is versatile in the sense that you can do many different exercises with it. The problem, as with most home equipment, is that none of the exercises you can do on it are as good as those performed on commercial-grade equipment found in nearly every gym in the country. And all the other negatives I mentioned about training at home apply here as well.
- **Almost anything promoted on an infomercial**, especially by these guys who pitch a different piece of equipment every few months. These guys – and you probably know who I'm talking about – have no shame. I must admit that they are good at making slick infomercials, but that's more than I can say about the exercise equipment they hawk. The problem is two-fold: The equipment they endorse is either of low quality, or is ineffective, or both. And, if each piece of equipment they sell is supposed to revolutionize the fitness world, why do they continue to come out with new stuff every few months?

Trendy Training Programs

Here I want to examine and give my analysis of some of the more popular training programs out there today.

Crossfit

During the last decade, crossfit has emerged as one of the most popular training approaches in the fitness arena. Crossfit combines various training methodologies into a holistic approach to improve fitness and athletic performance. The best way I can describe it is its attempt to combine strength and cardio work into every exercise performed and to complete a specific amount of work in a given period of time. Trainers either perform a lot of reps with relatively light weight or very few reps with heavy weight. The program features bodyweight and other exercises involving other unconventional (functional) movements. Many of the movements resemble those seen at Strong Man events – tire flips and carrying sandbags and other objects for a predetermined distance, as examples. If you've ever watched the Strong Man competitions, you'll notice that they lift heavy things, but they always have to see who gets the most reps or completes the task in the least amount of time. Crossfit is very similar in that there's always an element of endurance combined with feats of strength.

Due to its increased popularity, crossfit and "garage" gyms are popping up everywhere. Despite its popularity, I still group crossfit in with other fitness fads, once again keeping in mind that not all fads are necessarily bad. No doubt you can improve your fitness with crossfit, but I have some problems with it. The program, in my opinion, overemphasizes athletic performance at the expense of muscular hypertrophy. Most people don't compete in athletic events, and those who do, do so mainly for fun and recreation. So, developing athletic prowess should not be the primary purpose of a fitness program. Competitive athletes are athletes primarily because they already excel at the sport they compete in. Their training programs are generally very specific and designed to augment the skills and movements specific to their sport.

Crossfit combines aerobic and anaerobic training in all facets of training in an attempt to ramp up metabolic conditioning. This is good practice, in theory, as the trainee can get a great amount of work done in a relatively short span of time. This type of training is good for those wanting to lose weight, for example. The problem with relying on this type of training too much is that, once again, muscular hypertrophy is sacrificed. Research has clearly shown that aerobic training combined with weight training hinders muscular hypertrophy, and to some extent, vice-versa.

Part of the allure of crossfit is the competition among trainees as they try to beat one another's times to finish workouts. Trying to always beat the clock, though, encourages trainees to throw weights around in a rush, which may cause a breakdown in form and thus may contribute to injury. As one pushes their body to the max, fatigue sets in, and can also contribute to injury.

The workouts can be very demanding, which is usually a good thing. However, it may be too demanding for many, and certainly too demanding for someone simply seeking to improve their current level of fitness, not be a competitive athlete. For this reason, many people will not stick with progressively harder workouts.

Finally, crossfit can be very expensive, compared to many other fitness opportunities, including commercial gyms. From what I've seen, a membership at one of these franchised crossfit clubs ranges anywhere from around $60 to as much as $120 a month, whereas a commercial gym membership ranges from around $40 to $60 a month. For me, there's no comparison between the two. With a commercial gym membership, you get a full range of resistance and cardio machines, free weights, and other amenities like a pool and sauna. Many commercial gyms now have much of the equipment used in crossfit. If you go with a crossfit facility, you pay more for much less. Crossfit facilities commonly have ropes, rings, a few barbells, kettlebells, maybe some oversized tires, sandbags, and what have you. People join a crossfit facility to do crossfit exclusively. Some will argue that it's the experience that they are paying extra for. I, however, like to have a wide variety of equipment and the flexibility to structure my own workout, to work out alone if I want to, and to work out when I want to. Crossfit facilities do not give the trainee nearly as much flexibility, as their whole training program is centered around group training, at a set time, and performing a fixed workout (often called the WOD, workout of the day). In my view, the best way to incorporate crossfit into your fitness program is through periodization. In other words, engage in crossfit a few weeks at a time throughout the year as a change of pace to your regular training.

In summary, following a crossfit training regimen can certainly help someone improve their level of fitness, including fat loss and some gains in muscle. However, taking into account the issues I've discussed, it doesn't make sense to choose crossfit over a more traditional training program that one could employ at any commercial gym. If you want to try crossfit, incorporate some of its exercises into your regular routine, or once in a while, change things up by doing a crossfit workout. In other words, I believe that crossfit methodology can certainly be incorporated into anyone's training regimen. One should not, however, rely solely on crossfit to attain their fitness goals. It's too expensive, too restrictive (time and group training), and too demanding for most people, which contributes to injury and burnout.

P90X

P90X is an intense, 90-day training program that is done at home. For $120 consumers get a set of 12 DVDs that take trainees through the workouts. Also included are a fitness guide, a nutrition plan, and a calendar to track progress. P90X has been heavily marketed primarily through an effective infomercial and by word of mouth, which has been mostly positive. One of the program's selling points is that it employs a concept called muscle confusion. This means that the trainee is subjected to new exercises on a regular basis so that one's muscles can never fully adapt to the workout. P90X features strength training, cardio, plyometrics, yoga, and stretching. Strength training consists of body-weight movements, dumbbell exercises, and pull-ups.

P90X Pros and Cons

Many people have experienced good results with P90X, but there's nothing magical or even profound about the reasons for success. If you exercise intensely for an hour and a half each day and cut your caloric intake below maintenance, you will lose weight, guaranteed. My biggest problem with the program is that, like crossfit, it relies too much on aerobic exercise and not enough on resistance work. The resistance work that one does do is too low in intensity to build any appreciable muscle. It could be argued that people who are new to resistance training may gain some muscle, due to the fact that their muscles are responding to completely new stimuli. However, if you look at the individuals who have completed the program, most show some fat loss, which does aid in appearance (muscle tone) and fitness, but very few gain much muscle. And, like crossfit, the workouts can be extremely demanding, especially for beginners or those seeking only minor improvements.

In addition, plyometrics, which is high-impact training, can be very hard on the knees, feet, and lower back. For me, training at home is another disadvantage, since there are so many distractions at home. You also have to purchase some auxiliary equipment, like dumbbells, resistance bands, and a pull-up bar. P90X reminds me of the calisthenics I used to do in the Army – constant movement utilizing a wide variety of exercises for about an hour or so. The program provides the trainee a great deal of variety, challenge, and encouragement. Still, those with the most dedication experience the most success. The majority of people who begin the program don't finish. And then, what happens after the 90 days? Do people revert back to their old habits? An effective exercise plan should be ingrained in one's life, a lifestyle. For the most part, exercise should be enjoyable, not painstaking or drudgery. You should look forward to your workouts and feel good during and afterwards.

Insanity

The name says it all. Insanity is an intense, 60-day, home workout program. Like P90X, Insanity features highly intense workouts contained on 10 DVDs. Insanity features interval training consisting primarily of plyometrics combined with calisthenics and kick-boxing moves. The problems I have with P90X also apply to Insanity. I may be even less impressed with Insanity, due to the fact that it has trainees do fewer strength exercises than does P90X. There's no doubt that Insanity can deliver results for those who commit themselves to the program and watch what and how much they eat. However, like P90X, weight loss will be the primary outcome, with no appreciable gain in muscle. If weight loss and increased muscle tone is your only goal, then programs like Insanity and P90X will do the job. On the flip side, these types of high-intensity, high-impact programs are extremely challenging and not for the faint of heart.

I think these types of programs are popular today for several reasons:

- **Slick marketing**: Infomercials get better and better at suspending our critical thinking skills.
- **The impact of social media**: Word of mouth is now spread far and wide and instantaneously through social media such as YouTube and Facebook.
- **Something new**: People are desperate for something novel, even though these so called "new" programs are simply repackaged programs from the past.
- **Convenience of training at home**: Not everyone enjoys the gym experience as much as I do. There are some advantages to training at home: no wasted time in traffic getting to the gym; no waiting on equipment at the gym; no one watching you during your workout.

The Biggest Diet Fads

Since almost everyone is trying to lose weight, at one time or another, people are always looking for the latest diet that promises to take the weight off and keep it off. In fact, many diet books have been on the best-selling lists, with many achieving cult-like status. As with other fitness trends, a fad diet that gains popularity is not necessarily bad. However, as with all fads, diets come and go, which tells me that there is no single best diet. There certainly is no magic diet, no unique combination of foods or macronutrients that cause you to lose weight without cutting calories below maintenance for an extended period of time. In essence, all diets work, if they require you to take in fewer calories than you use and you follow the program. Fad diets are likely to remain popular as people desperately seek quick and easy answers to weight loss.

- **Atkins**: Arguably, the most popular diet book and fad of all time. Low-carb diets have come and gone for a long time, but Dr. Atkins' book changed the diet culture. Still somewhat popular, for a few years in the late 90's and early into the past decade, all you heard was low carbs. The premise of the diet is that by cutting out most carbs, the body has to pull more readily from its fat stores for energy. This process does happen, and the diet does work, but only because you are creating a caloric deficit. And the downsides are that you have to eat a lot of fat and eliminate most healthful fruits and vegetables, both of which are unhealthy over time.

- **Blood Type**: This diet claims that we should eat or not eat certain foods based on your individual blood type. Most nutrition experts dismiss it due to a general lack of scientific support.
- **Cabbage Soup**: This diet comes and goes with regularity. The idea is to eat a lot of cabbage soup for a couple of weeks and not much else. The diet definitely works, as dieters are able to lose weight quickly. But eating cabbage soup every day gets old real fast, and any lost weight is quickly regained as soon as you start eating real food again.
- **Detox**: There are many detox plans out there. Detoxing has become all the rage in Hollywood, as a way to drop weight very quickly, and the most popular detox diet currently out there is the Hollywood 48-hour Miracle Diet. The idea behind detoxing is that we need to cleanse the body periodically by ridding it of toxins. This process usually consists of either fasting for a while or fasting with certain juices, other liquids, and vitamins. There's very little science showing that you can actually detoxify the body through dietary means, or that the body even needs, or somehow benefits from, detoxification. Moreover, extended fasting can be dangerous, and is certainly not healthful.
- **Dukan**: Named after the French doctor who created it, the Dukan Diet is another very low-carb diet. It is similar to the Atkins Diet, but Dukan emphasizes high protein and relatively low fat.
- **Glycemic Index**: The glycemic index ranks carbs on how fast they convert to glucose once eaten. The faster, the higher score. Carbs that convert quickly to glucose cause a big spike in insulin, which can cause greater fat storage. The diet emphasizes avoiding high glycemic carbs and instead eating primarily mid-to-low glycemic carbs. The problem is that eating proteins and fats with carbs alters the rate at which they convert to glucose.
- **Grapefruit**: People have been pushing grapefruit as a fat emulsifier for a long time. Presumably, people believe that there is some special ingredient – an enzyme or something – that magically burns fat. Eat one grapefruit a day, at breakfast, and lose weight. Grapefruit is very nutritious, but has not been shown, by itself, to cause weight loss. On the other hand, eating grapefruit while lowering calories below maintenance has been shown to cause

weight loss.

- **Fasting**: Fasting is still a common approach to weight loss. Not eating will cause rapid weight loss, but it becomes very unhealthy the longer you do it. Short fasts, of no longer than a day and done infrequently, are considered safe and may even be healthy.
- **HCG**: HCG is human chorionic gonadotropin, a hormone produced during pregnancy and is mainly used to treat fertility issues. There is no evidence that HCG helps people lose weight. What's worse, HCG has not even been approved for over-the-counter sale. So what is actually being sold in stores or online? On top of that, the diet restricts calories to between 500 and 1,000 a day. One is likely to lose weight on so few calories, but it's very unlikely that HCG does anything, if, in fact, there is any real HCG in the product.
- **Low-Fat**: Long before the low-carb craze, there was the low-fat craze, when everything was low fat. Everyone went around counting how many fat grams they were consuming with everything they ate. Several popular diets came out of this era and helped fuel the low-fat movement. The top three, in my opinion were the T-Factor, Ornish, and Pritikin Diets. The main idea is that because fat has more energy than protein or carbs, one can more easily control caloric (energy) consumption by decreasing fat intake. Doctors argued that by limiting fat intake, especially saturated fat, one could reduce cholesterol and stave off heart disease. The low-fat diets have shown some promise in this area, but the primary problem is getting people to stick to them. And now we know that we need to eat more good fats while limiting bad fats.
- **Paleo**: Often called the "Caveman" diet, this diet tries to emulate what hunter-gatherers of the Paleolithic era would have eaten, prior to the agricultural age. The diet, therefore, includes fish, lean meats, eggs, fruits, vegetables, roots, and nuts and excludes dairy, potatoes, grains, legumes, refined sugar, and processed oils. Advocates claim that early humans became well adapted to this type of diet and that modern humans are not well adapted to what we currently eat. This current mal-adaption, they claim, is the leading cause of obesity and other diseases, like heart disease. The Paleo Diet can help fight obesity, but the claims about preventing heart disease seem to be unfounded. As it turns out, scans of mummified bodies from the Paleolithic era clearly show that people of that era had developed hardening of the arteries, the same as people do today.
- **Protein Power**: Very similar to Atkins but with a bit more

emphasis on protein and less on fat. This book went a long way in calling attention to the importance of eating substantial protein while dieting. The emphasis on low carbs, though, leaves it open to the same criticisms that apply to all low-carb diets, with the main ones being a lack of important nutrients contained in many carb food sources and that it's boring and difficult to follow.

- **South Beach**: The main difference with this diet is its emphasis on choosing good carbs and fats over bad ones. Good carbs are those low on the glycemic index, and good fats are unsaturated and high in omega-3 fatty acids.
- **The Zone**: The "Zone" is when the hormones insulin and glucagon are in the proper balance. According to Dr. Barry Sears, this balance is best achieved when eating carbs, protein, and fat in a 40:30:30 ratio. Sears also argues that this particular macronutrient ratio helps to alleviate inflammation in the body. Due to the Zone's attention to eating and supplementing more omega-3 and omega-6 oil, Sears is widely credited with starting this healthful trend within the general population.

- **Weight Loss Systems**: The biggies out there are, of course, Weight Watchers, Nutrisystem, and Jenny Craig. Weight Watchers uses a point system for foods, and you try not to exceed your daily allotment of points. Weight Watchers is, essentially, a support group, and dieters meet regularly to discuss their progress and struggles. Nutrisystem and Jenny Craig both feature pre-packaged meals that are delivered directly to their clients. Pre-packaged meals makes it easier to eat only what is in front of you, and you know exactly the caloric and nutrient content of what you are eating.

Perspective

The bottom line is that there is no shortage of diets or nutrition plans out there, and they all work to some extent. I have a strong suspicion, though, that it's not a particular diet that does the trick, but simply reducing total calories. I'm not against someone following a fad diet, if it meets your needs. But, on the other hand, I'd like for us to get away from diets altogether and begin to think about lifelong nutrition. That means adopting a long-term instead of a short-term approach to weight management. Nutrition is extremely important, but it is only part of a bigger picture that makes up a fitness lifestyle.

10. NUTRITION BASICS

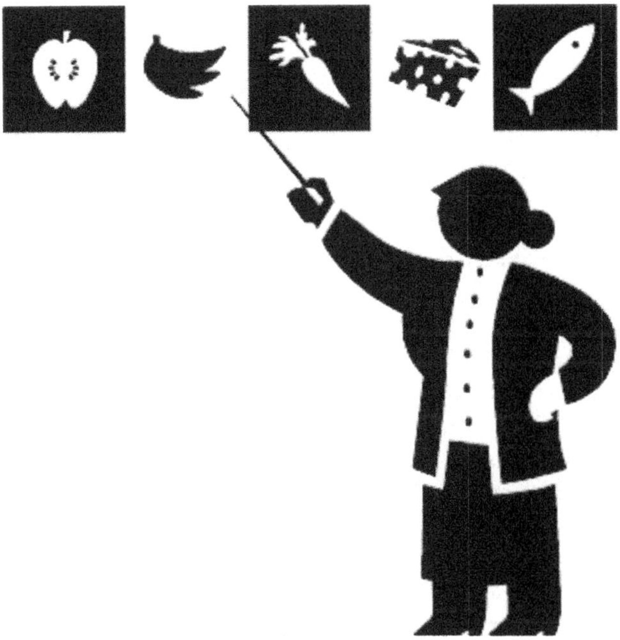

People say that losing weight is no walk in the park. When I hear that I think, yeah, that's the problem. – Chris Adams

I want to disclose right up front that I'm not a medical doctor nor do I have a degree in nutrition. I'm not an expert on nutrition, by way of credentials. My knowledge of nutrition comes from my personal experience, including all that I've read and studied, which is voluminous. Most diet books – many of which are fads – are written by physicians or nutritionists. However, many of these authors and their books are responsible for the majority of diet fads we see today. My point is that just because someone has credentials doesn't necessarily mean that you should buy into everything they say about diet and nutrition. Since I am not an expert – at least not as far as credentials – my goal is to present nutrition information that is backed up by scientific consensus. I will also share my own personal experience regarding nutrition strategies.

Even in today's information age, nutrition is a hodgepodge of myths, misconceptions, and misinformation. There's been thousands of diet books published over the past couple of decades, and fads rule the day. Nutrition science isn't much better, as studies contradict one another. Nutrition experts warn us that certain foods are bad for us, only to turn around a few years later to give their okay to the very foods that they warned us about. It's no wonder that people are confused about what to eat.

With all the confusion out there, how are we supposed to figure out which foods we should eat and which ones we should avoid? Obviously, we can't rely on the results of one study to base our food choices on. Rather, we must consider the cumulative data from many studies. This means that we have to be critical thinkers. We have to weigh various sources of information and judge for ourselves whom and what to believe. Therefore, it's up to each of us to be as well informed as possible about our own food choices. It's important to read all you can about nutrition and keep an open mind. And when in doubt, use common sense.

There is good news in all this confusion. While there is still much debate about preferred food choices and dietary strategies, the science of weight gain and weight loss is well grounded in basic physics, and the laws of physics cannot be violated. In this area there is no mystery, no magic. No matter what some doctors or nutritional experts might say to the contrary, weight loss and weight gain depends upon your energy consumption versus energy expenditure. Your body stores extra consumed energy as fat. This simple energy equation gives us a guide to go by: calories in versus calories out.

Why is Losing Fat So Difficult?

If it weren't for the fact that the TV set and the refrigerator are so far apart, some of us wouldn't get any exercise at all. – Joey Adams

The primary reason that losing fat is so difficult is because, over the course of human evolution, our bodies became very efficient at storing fat, an effective survival adaptation to help us endure famines, which were quite common until only recently in our history. Once again, the law of conservation of energy comes into play, and in a big way. In our past, energy, whether in the form of food or stored fat, was extremely valuable and something to be used very judiciously. Why would someone expend valuable energy running around for no good reason? Most of the energy we expended was to gather more energy, as in hunting and gathering food. It seems obvious that these survival behaviors became part of our genetic makeup and are still with us today. Another part of our genetic makeup – our craving for high-fat, high-calorie foods – makes it that much more difficult for us to lose unwanted fat.

When you think about it, denying yourself food as an attempt to lose weight is really a bizarre behavior for any species. In fact, for most species we equate fatness with fitness. Most of human history has been about getting enough to eat, not trying to lose weight. Today, of course, we are victims of our own prosperity by being surrounded with too many high-calorie, processed foods, and which are too easy to get and consume. Further compounding the problem, our postmodern lifestyle doesn't require, or even encourage, us to move nearly enough, and therefore we don't expend enough calories in our day-to-day lives. This type of environment in which we find ourselves is truly a recipe for disaster. So, I hate to be so brief and concise, but it's no great mystery. We keep getting fatter due to just a few key developments, and all of them have to do with technology and our postmodern lifestyle:

- We consume too much processed food, which is loaded with chemicals, sodium, bad fats, and sugars, and which often has most of the fiber removed.
- We consume way too much fast food, which is loaded with calories, bad fats, and sodium.
- We eat way too much of the wrong foods – too much of the above and not enough fruits and vegetables in their natural state.
- We don't get nearly enough exercise. Most of us have sedentary jobs and do not get enough exercise on our own.

Some experts claim that we actually consume fewer calories today than we did in 1960, but I have a hard time believing this. Have you watched people navigate a buffet lately? It's as if these people haven't eaten in days, or they are about to consume their last meal and thus don't want to leave anything out. Of course, with the amount and type of greasy food some of these porkers chow down on, it might very well be their last meal. In addition to buffets, people eat out more often than in the past, and portions have steadily become larger. Much of the food we eat today is produced and packaged for our convenience. The problem is that most of these convenience foods are calorically dense and loaded with sugar, sodium, and a ton of preservatives. Our food has become so easy to get and prepare. We used to have to hunt, gather, or grow our food. Now we are literally drowning in food, but, unfortunately, so much of it is bad for us, and makes losing fat and keeping it off nearly impossible.

Some lay all of the blame for the precipitous rise in obesity rates on our consumption of sugar, and especially high fructose corn syrup (HFCS). HFCS is cheaper than plain cane sugar, so companies have virtually replaced sugar with it in most products, and it is everywhere. We certainly do consume a lot of this stuff, and it is no doubt a contributor to the problem, but it can't be blamed for all of our weight gain. HFCS does cause a spike in insulin. A major function of insulin is to help the body deal with sugar by shuttling it into muscles and the liver in the form of glycogen. Insulin also converts extra sugar into triglycerides to be stored as fat. The degree to which a food causes insulin to spike is called the glycemic index. Some carbohydrates cause insulin to spike quickly and thus causes blood glucose levels to rise quickly in response and remain more unstable as the body attempts to deal with every infusion of carbohydrates. This has prompted the low-carb diet frenzy, and more recently, the low-glycemic index diet. Many feel that any foods that cause a spike in insulin are potentially more fattening than foods that leave glucose levels relatively stable. This process, though, has many variables, one of which is the total amount of calories in the food and the fact that foods are usually mixed in any given meal.

Studies consistently show that the total number of calories we consume is the primary determinate of whether we gain or lose weight. And here I use "weight" in place of fat, since when we gain or lose weight we also gain or lose muscle and/or water. The first law of thermodynamics – the law of conservation of energy – states that energy cannot be created or destroyed, only transformed. The energy consumed via food is transformed into energy that fuels the body. Excess energy we consume is transformed into fat which is stored in the body. A calorie really is a calorie. However, we all don't burn calories at the same rate. That's why some people can eat more and remain thin while others eat less but remain fat.

To illustrate my point about total calories, a food scientist recently lost 27 pounds during an 8-week period by eating mostly junk food, most of it laden with sugar and HFCS. He ate approximately 1,800 calories a day, and did not exercise a great deal. In addition to the weight loss, some key indicators of health – like total cholesterol and triglycerides – actually improved. I don't recommend that you emulate his food choices, but he did prove an important point: Total calorie intake matters more in weight loss than the composition of the calories.

What's the Best Way to Lose Fat?

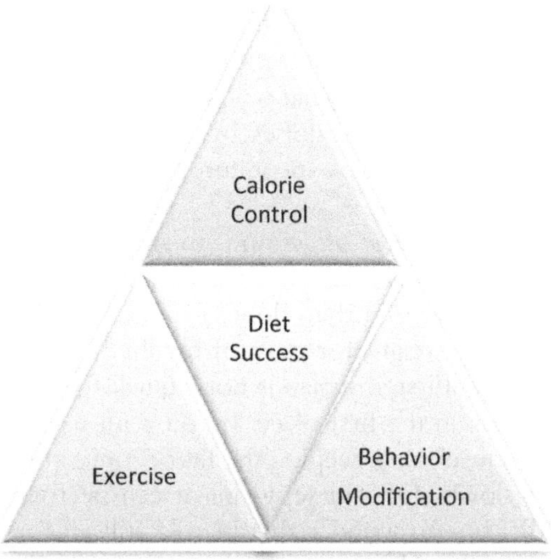

The only approach to fat loss that has been shown to work over the long term is a multi-faceted approach involving calorie control, regular exercise, and behavior modification, as depicted in the triangle above. To lose fat and not muscle, one must create a caloric deficit, but just barely. In other words, you must take in fewer calories but not to the extent that your body interprets it as starvation. If you cut back too far on calorie intake, your metabolism will slow drastically to help maintain its fat reserves. Under severe caloric restrictions your body will actually eat its own muscle, metabolizing amino acids for energy. To retain as much muscle mass as possible, you must engage in heavy resistance work. If you can add muscle, you will end up burning more calories, even at rest, due to the metabolic demands of muscle. In addition to intense resistance work, one must simply move more, which could be any kind of movement . . . walking, gardening, housework, etc. Burning calories through exercise – any sort of exercise – helps to create a caloric deficit. Many people don't help themselves by always taking the easy way. People should pick up habits of moving more whenever they have the choice, like taking the stairs instead of the elevator, for example, or parking at the back of the parking lot so you'll have to walk farther. These habits are not insignificant; they can add up over time. Moreover, they form the basis of a more healthy and fitness-conscious lifestyle.

Many people have the misguided notion that they can eat more than they should if they exercise enough to "work it off." The problem is that people don't burn off nearly as many calories while exercising as they think they do. The average person, for example, burns only about 100 calories during a one-mile walk. One plain donut has more than twice that many calories. So, for most people, it is unreasonable to think that they can make up for what they eat with exercise. It makes more sense to simply pass on the donut . . . and the walk. Of course, the best thing would be to pass on the donut and walk for an hour. That would be the most reasonable way to create a caloric deficit . . . cut calories by about 10 to 20 percent below maintenance and increase caloric expenditure through exercise by about 200 – 300 per day.

So, by far, the best course of action is to simply eat a little bit less and exercise a lot more, with a big part of the exercise being resistance training. I realize that this is easier said than done. I know this all too well, since I have struggled with my weight for most of my life. I should warn you of a couple of caveats here: First, my plan is not a quick fix, as quick fixes never last, even if they work in the first place. If you want to have any chance of holding onto your muscle and keeping the fat off once you lose it, then you must lose the fat slowly. Of course, losing it can be frustrating, since we want it off ASAP. It's no wonder that people still go for the quick fixes, even though none of them have ever produced lasting effects.

In terms of macronutrients, I prefer something close to the following distribution: 40 percent carbohydrates, 30 percent protein, and 30 percent fat, as put forward in the Zone Diet by Dr. Barry Sears. The "Zone" is when the hormones insulin and glucagon are in the proper balance. According to Dr. Sears, this balance is best achieved when eating carbs, protein, and fat in a 40:30:30 ratio. Sears also argues that this particular macronutrient ratio helps to alleviate inflammation in the body. I'm not claiming that there's something magical about this particular ratio, which, if you follow it, will cause you lose more fat than other ratios of macronutrients. It does, however, allow me to eat many of the foods I like.

However you structure your diet, the most important thing to remember is that you absolutely must create a caloric deficit in order to lose fat, regardless of the proportions of macronutrients. The 40:30:30 proportion works best for me because it meets my body's training needs and is something I can stick to. There are good and bad carbs, and the same is true for fats and proteins. The trick is to eat mainly the good choices from each group while limiting the bad ones. With carbs, I limit high-glycemic carbs while eating more higher-fiber ones. High-glycemic carbs spike insulin levels, which can contribute to fat gain, since helping the body store fat is one of the functions of insulin. Spikes in insulin are usually followed by drastic drops in blood sugar levels, which brings on hunger again. See the table below for a list of the relative glycemic index of selected carbs. The glycemic load (gl) might be a better indicator of good and bad carbs, since it takes the total grams of carbohydrate per serving into consideration. Keep in mind that carbs are usually eaten with proteins and fats, which can alter the rate in which they get converted into glucose.

GI and GL for Common Foods				
Food	GI	Serving Size	Net Carbs	GL
Peanuts	14	4 oz (113g)	15	2
Bean sprouts	25	1 cup (104g)	4	1
Grapefruit	25	1/2 large (166g)	11	3
Pizza	30	2 slices (260g)	42	13
Lowfat yogurt	33	1 cup (245g)	47	16
Apples	38	1 medium (138g)	16	6
Spaghetti	42	1 cup (140g)	38	16
Carrots	47	1 large (72g)	5	2
Oranges	48	1 medium (131g)	12	6
Bananas	52	1 large (136g)	27	14
Potato chips	54	4 oz (114g)	55	30
Snickers Bar	55	1 bar (113g)	64	35
Brown rice	55	1 cup (195g)	42	23
Honey	55	1 tbsp (21g)	17	9
Oatmeal	58	1 cup (234g)	21	12
Ice cream	61	1 cup (72g)	16	10
Macaroni and cheese	64	1 serving (166g)	47	30
Raisins	64	1 small box (43g)	32	20
White rice	64	1 cup (186g)	52	33
Sugar (sucrose)	68	1 tbsp (12g)	12	8
White bread	70	1 slice (30g)	14	10
Watermelon	72	1 cup (154g)	11	8
Popcorn	72	2 cups (16g)	10	7
Baked potato	85	1 medium (173g)	33	28
Glucose	100	(50g)	50	50

With protein, I try to eat more lean choices like lean red meat, chicken breast and fish. Many people shun eggs because of the high amount of cholesterol contained in the yolk. There's no need to fear, since the cholesterol in foods has little impact on the total cholesterol level in our body. Moreover, egg yolks contain lecithin, vitamin B12, and healthy omega-3 fatty acids. I drink about 10-12 ounces of milk a day, and I prefer 2 percent fat. About the only other dairy product I consume on a regular basis is cheese. There virtually no food that can't be made better by putting cheese on it. Don't neglect the protein content of vegetables, legumes, and whole grains. Legumes, like many beans, are loaded with protein and high in fiber.

Like with carbs and protein, there are definitely good and bad fats. I try to eat foods high in essential fatty acids, like omega 3, which are found in fish, nuts, and olive oil. I also supplement my diet with fish and flax seed oil caplets. Trans fats, the very bad fats, should be avoided at all costs, as these fats have been altered (hydrogenated) by production processes to last longer on the shelf. The problem is that the hydrogenation process that alters the fat molecules makes the fat harmful to our bodies, especially our blood vessels. Read the ingredient list of processed foods and you'll find that most of them contained some sort of either "hydrogenated" or "partially hydrogenated" oil. That's one reason why so many processed foods are unhealthy and should be avoided or at least kept to a minimum.

I eat basically three meals a day with two additional snacks spaced in between. My goal is to never get too hungry. When I get too hungry, I end up overeating. While I try to eat healthy, I still eat whatever I want, just not how much I want. People shouldn't deprive themselves. If you go too strict with your diet, you are more likely to binge. And food brings us so much pleasure in life. Why deprive yourself of the food you love, just eat less of it. That's one of the main problems with many of the fad diets. They require dieters to restrict or completely eliminate many of the foods they love the most. And that's why they fail. People simply cannot stick to them for very long. Losing and maintaining a healthy weight is more than blindly following a diet; it's about adopting a nutritional plan that you can live with and be happy. Moreover, it's a lifestyle that involves healthy eating and exercise.

My Own Diet

It's difficult to lay out what I eat on a daily basis, since I eat a wide variety of foods. Here is simply an example of what I eat on a typical day, along with the nutrient content.

Example of My Daily Food Intake				
Food	**Calories**	**Macronutrients**		
Breakfast		**Carbs**	**Protein**	**Fat**
Egg McMuffin	300	30	18	12
1 Cup 2% Milk	122	12	8	5
1 Piece of Fruit	90	21	1	0
Totals	512	63	27	17
Lunch				
Grilled Chicken Breast	230	0	43	6
Serving of Rice or Baked Potato	130	25	5	1
Green Vegetable	60	13	3	0
Small Piece of Candy	60	5	1	4

Diet Soda	0	0	0	0
Totals	480	43	52	11
Dinner				
1 Hamburger Patty or Piece of Sirloin	250	0	33	13
Serving of Mashed Potatoes or Sweet Potato	120	24	4	1
Small Tossed Salad or Cole Slaw	150	16	4	8
Small Dessert	200	27	2	9
Totals	720	67	43	31
Snacks				
Beef Jerky	90	7	13	1
String Cheese	110	2	7	8
Protein Bar	300	29	30	7
Totals	500	38	50	16
Grand Totals	2,212	194	172	75

If you do the math on the grand daily total, you will see that it is very close to the 40:30:30 ratio I mentioned previously. In this particular example, the exact ratio is 38 percent carbs, 31 percent protein, and 31 percent fat. About once a week I have a cheat day, where I consume an additional 400-500 calories over maintenance. These additional calories come largely from carbohydrates, as in a stack of pancakes and syrup, for example. Then some days I stay below maintenance in caloric intake. So, things tend to balance out over the course of the week. I pay more attention to overall calories than the ratio of the individual macronutrients. At the end of the day, maintenance of one's weight comes down to calories in, calories out. I'm able to stay close to the 40:30:30 ratio because of the eating habits I've developed and my individual food preferences.

Nutrition Myths That Just Won't Die

With all the research into diet and nutrition, you would think that the public would be well informed on the subject, but it seems that nothing is further from the truth. Nutrition myths hold on because people keep believing them and passing them on, even in the face of research data. Here are some of the more popular myths:

- **You must drink 8-10 glasses of water each day**. Obviously, we need a certain amount of water to survive. However, that amount varies greatly among individuals and is influenced by our activities and especially by how much we sweat in a given period of time. How much water you need is dependent on how much total fluid you consume in the form of other beverages, like milk, soda, coffee, etc. As a general rule, drink when you are thirsty and drink more immediately before, during, and after your workouts, especially if you sweat a lot.

- **Drinking ice water helps you lose weight by speeding up your metabolism**. The idea here is that your stomach/intestines have to warm the cold water, thereby making more work for your body. But, seriously, how long does it take for that water you drink to warm up to the temperature of your body. It isn't long and your body barely notices it.
- **Eggs will raise your cholesterol**. Since the yolk contains a lot of cholesterol, doctors told their patients with high cholesterol to avoid eggs. However, studies have confirmed that even people being treated for high cholesterol can eat up to seven eggs a week without raising their total cholesterol levels significantly.
- **Eating at night will make you fat**. People still believe that since you don't burn as many calories while sleeping, food eaten late in the day is more likely to be stored as fat. The only important thing, though, is how many total calories you consume over a period of time.
- **Breakfast is the most important meal of the day**. I know this is nutrition heresy, but breakfast is somewhat overrated. Studies do show that those who eat breakfast regularly weigh less than those who don't. So we've had it drilled into our heads that we must start the day with breakfast or our day will be ruined, we'll gain weight, and we'll be unhealthy. Many people, however, simply aren't hungry until they've been up for a while. For them, eating breakfast only adds calories when they aren't even motivated to eat. You shouldn't eat until you are hungry. For many, then, brunch is the most important meal of the day.
- **Vitamin supplements are necessary for optimum health**. People think that taking vitamin supplements will give them more energy and make them healthier. There's no evidence that this is the case. Eating an unhealthy diet – one that doesn't provide enough nutrients – can lead to vitamin and mineral deficiencies, which can impair one's health. This condition is relatively rare in the developed world. Apparently, although many Americans eat a relatively unhealthy diet, we eat enough food to make up for it.

- **Eating immediately after a workout will improve recovery**. This mantra is common in muscle and fitness magazines. The theory is that immediately after a hard workout (a resistance-dominated workout), it is important to replenish your glycogen stores in muscles, and this surge of simple carbs spikes insulin, which drives amino acids into muscle cells. The amino acids are contained in the protein shake you are required to drink immediately after your workout. There's conflicting studies showing that consuming a high-protein meal or shake immediately after a workout contributes to, or does not contribute to, enhanced muscular hypertrophy or general recovery.
- **You need a lot more protein to build muscle**. This one has been around for a long time. To build muscle you do need a little more protein, but you need more carbs and fat, too. In other words, to build more muscle, you simply need more calories. Building muscle requires energy, and that energy has to come from somewhere. Protein gets pushed so much because it is big business among supplement companies.
- **Carbohydrates make you fat**. The low-carb craze has pretty much run its course, thank goodness. Your brain runs solely on carbohydrates. Want to feel and act like a zombie? Go low carbs for a few days. Most of the foods that are good for you are carbohydrates. You can't possibly get all of the nutrients your body needs without eating a significant amount of your daily calories from carbohydrates. There are some carbs that should be limited. I'm talking about most simple carbs, like sugar, sugar-laden sweets – like soda, cookies, muffins, etc. – and foods containing white, refined flour. These carbs do contribute more to weight gain, due primarily to their impact on insulin, lack of fiber, and dearth of nutrients.
- **High-fructose corn syrup is worse for you than sucrose.** Structurally, they're not that different. I think HFCS has been especially demonized because it is in virtually everything we eat. Because it is so cheap, it has replaced sugar in the foods we eat.
- **Sea salt is healthier than regular salt**. No evidence that it is, and regular salt has iodine, which prevents goiter.
- **Organic foods are healthier than regular foods**. Studies have not shown organic foods to be any healthier than regular foods. You might want to consume organic foods for ethical reasons, but don't expect them to make you any healthier.
- **Eating smaller more frequent meals is better than eating three larger meals.** People claim that smaller, more frequent

meals helps to better regulate blood sugar levels and thus keeps you from getting too hungry between meals and overeating. This sounds good, but there is little actual research to support it. In fact, most of the research supports the traditional three-meal a day approach. Larger meals tend to fill you up and satisfy you more than smaller meals. Some studies have even shown not much difference in weight loss or performance, regardless of the number of meals eaten on a daily basis.

Dietary Recommendations That Make Sense

- Eat a wide variety of foods, and base your diet around fresh foods and vegetables.
- Eat more whole grains like whole grain breads, pasta and rice, which have more fiber than their processed counterparts.
- Eat lean meat selections for protein.
- Eat more fish for lean protein and omega-3 fatty acids.
- Limit processed sugars while eating more natural sugars, like most fruits.
- Eat three meals a day with healthy snacks in between, if desired.

Foods You Should Eat More Often

The Most Healthful Foods			
Veggies	**Fruits**	**Grains**	**Beans**
Asparagus	Apples	Barley	Black Beans
Broccoli	Blueberries	Brown Rice	Garbanzo Beans
Carrots	Cranberries	Buckwheat	Kidney Beans
Celery	Grapefruit	Corn	Lima Beans
Kale	Oranges	Millet	Miso
Onions	Pears	Oats	Navy Beans
Spinach	Plums	Quinoa	Pinto Beans
Squash	Raspberries	Rye	Soybeans
Sweet Potatoes	Strawberries	Spelt	Tempeh
Tomatoes	Watermelon	Whole Wheat	Tofu

The Most Healthful Foods – Continued			
Nuts	**Seafood**	**Drinks**	**Spices**
Almonds	Cod	Cranberry Juice	Basil
Cashews	Halibut	Fruit Smoothie	Cilantro
Flaxseeds	Mackerel	Green Tea	Ginger
Macadamia Nuts	Oysters	Low-fat Milk	Oregano
Peanuts	Salmon	Mint Tea	Parsley
Pistachios	Sardines	Orange Juice	Peppermint
Pumpkin Seeds	Scallops	Soy Milk	Rosemary
Sesame Seeds	Shrimp	Tomato Juice	Sage
Sunflower Seeds	Tilapia	Vegetable Juice	Thyme
Walnuts	Tuna	Water	Turmeric

Are Some Foods Off Limits?

Instead of completely ruling out certain foods, maybe we should say that there are foods that we should eat more often – like in the list above – and those we should eat less often. The old adage "all things in moderation" is especially apt when considering what and how much to eat. We might agree that particular foods are less healthful than others. That only means that we should eat less of those foods, not eliminate them altogether. In many cases, it's not the food itself that's unhealthy; it's how it is prepared or processed that does the damage. And as far as weight gain or loss, what you eat is not nearly as important as how much you eat. This has been shown to be true in research and numerous anecdotal examples. There are people who have, for example, lost a significant amount of weight while eating primarily fast food, and others while eating mainly snack cakes and candy bars. And then there are those who have gained weight while eating a diet composed primarily of foods commonly recognized as being healthful. We can't escape the fact that calories do matter, a lot. If you consume more calories than you burn, you will gain fat, no matter what you eat. Keeping this in mind, there are certain foods that we should eat sparingly, not simply because they may contribute to weight gain; they are simply not good for us, as they have been shown to contribute to non-fitness and disease.

Foods to Eat Sparingly

- **French Fries**: Undoubtedly, the worst thing you could do to a potato – deep fry it in oil and add copious amount of salt. Not good.
- **Soda**: 10 teaspoons of sugar per 12-ounce serving, not to mention a surfeit of preservatives, artificial flavorings, and dyes. Many

people could lose weight simply be cutting back on the amount of soda they drink.

- **Deep-Fried Foods**: French fries are only the beginning of this adulteration of food. Foods absorb the oils they are cooked in, which adds mega calories, and the fats become altered due to the cooking process.
- **Cake, Cookies, Candy, and Other Sweets**: The main problem with these, other than the high amount of sugar, is that they are devoid of any nutritional value. If that weren't reason enough to avoid them, many prepackaged gooey goodies are awash in trans fats, the type of fat that is particularly unhealthy.
- **Fast Food**: Most fast food is loaded with calories, saturated fat, and sodium. Some healthy choices do exist, but most people buckle under the temptation of the bad stuff. In a positive move, most restaurants now list the nutritional content of their food, so at least you know what you're getting. I find it best to simply steer clear of these places.
- **Processed Lunch Meats**: Loaded with sodium and preservatives, like nitrites. Nitrites have even been connected to an increased risk of colon cancer.
- **Solid Fats**: Fats that remain solid at room temperature are generally considered more unhealthy than liquid fats. On a related note, butter is better than margarine.
- **Chips and Other Salty Snacks**: Too high in fat and sodium and completely lacking any nutritional value. Baked versions are somewhat better, but still should be eaten sparingly.
- **White Refined Flour and Most Store-Bought Pasta**: All the good – the bran and germ – have been removed thus taking out all the fiber. A much better choice is whole wheat.
- **Whole Milk**: Too much fat and cholesterol. Skim is best. If that is too watery for you, try 1 percent. After a while you can get used to it.
- **Creamy Salad Dressings**: Read the labels. Most of these are extremely high in calories and saturated fat. I'm talking about 200 or more calories per serving, which is usually just a tablespoon. Who can enjoy a salad with only one tablespoon of salad dressing? So, people trying to lose weight think they are doing good by having a salad. But, more often than not, salads end up just as bad as other high-calorie, high-fat food. It's best to stick to the low-cal versions or good old oil and vinegar.

Fat Loss Habits

Adopting and sticking to sound dietary habits is the key to sustained weight loss. I know that this is easier said than done, but one has to try. And one has to start somewhere. Simply adopting a few healthful habits can make a huge difference over time. Here are some habits that will make a difference in your weight loss efforts:

- Portion control is the key. Calories must be cut back slightly below maintenance, while activity levels are increased significantly.
- Take a long-range approach instead of short-term. That way you're more likely to keep the fat off.
- Cut back on high-calorie, low-nutrition food choices, like sodas, sweet snacks, chips, etc.
- Avoid buffets like the plague. It's virtually impossible not to overeat at a buffet.
- Eat out less often and eat fast food even less than that.
- Eat smaller portions and only get seconds if you are truly still hungry. Often, one serving will fill you up.
- Make good/healthy food choices at the grocery. Don't bring home stuff that is going to sabotage your diet.
- Eat breakfast, or at least eat something nutritious early in the day. If you are not hungry first thing in the morning, then eat as soon as you feel hungry.
- Get in the habit of exercising every day, even if it's just a short walk or housework.

Supplements Worth Looking At

I do take a number of supplements on a regular basis, but let me say that I'm not a big fan of supplements. You can make good progress without taking any supplements. In fact, most of the supplements out there are next to worthless, or, at best, overhyped. I've been around the fitness world for a long time, so I've seen a lot of supplements come and go, and I've tried most of them. There are a few supplements out there that have risen above the others, due to the fact that they have some solid science behind them. Here are the supplements I currently take and can recommend.

- **Creatine**: A substance found naturally in muscle tissue, creatine is a critical component in the body's ATP production process. ATP (adenosine triphosphate) is what powers muscular contractions. When muscles are under extreme stress – like when lifting heavy weights for several reps – ATP is being used up quickly and must be replenished quickly. That's where creatine comes in. Creatine combines with phosphate to form phosphocreatine and can then replenish ATP stores. It has been shown that supplementing with creatine, at 5 grams a day, helps to replenish ATP stores faster and therefore can enable a lifter to carry a set further (do more reps). Creatine also hydrates muscle cells making them bigger and setting up an environment within the cell that contributes to anabolism. Creatine has been studied and tested more than any other supplement so far, and up to this point, it appears to be safe and devoid of any real side effects.

- Be aware that creatine comes in various forms, such as creatine monohydrate, phosphate, esters, or hydrochloride, with each claiming to be the best. All the research I have seen still places plain creatine monohydrate as being the most effective, and it is the least expensive of the lot. Many supplement companies still direct users of their creatine to load up on it when first starting on it. This means taking 20 grams a day for seven days and then taking 5 grams a day to maintain creatine levels in the body. There's really nothing wrong with this – other than being a bit wasteful – as research has shown that 5 grams a day from the very beginning of administration will saturate muscles with creatine at about the same rate as the higher dosage.

- **Multi-Vitamin/Mineral**: For as long as vitamin pills have been touted as health and energy boosters, there's very little scientific evidence to support these claims. On the contrary, recent studies have shown that supplementing certain vitamins actually puts you at a greater risk of developing certain diseases and dying sooner rather than extending life. One thing seems clear: it is best to get vitamins and minerals from their natural sources: food. This means it is vitally important to eat a well-balanced diet that supplies all of your nutritional needs. However, few people can pull this off. Add to that the reality that intense exercise places additional demands and stress upon the body. Because of this, I still believe that a daily multi-vitamin/mineral helps to ensure that people can meet their nutritional needs.

- **Caffeine**: Caffeine is the closest thing we have to a wonder drug. Many people could not function without their morning infusion of caffeine. Caffeine is in our sodas, energy drinks, weight-loss products, and even some aspirin formulas. Caffeine stimulates the central nervous system, which enhances alertness, strength, and endurance. For these reasons, many athletes take caffeine just prior to their workouts or athletic events. There's another important reason to supplement with caffeine before exercise. In addition to enhancing physical capabilities, caffeine also mobilizes fat so it can be burned as fuel during exercise.

People can become desensitized to caffeine, if it is overused, as in drinking several cups of coffee daily. Therefore, to get the maximum benefits of caffeine every workout, I use it very strategically. This means that I only take caffeine prior to my workouts, which is typically four days a week, and I don't drink coffee during the day. Just remember that caffeine is a drug and must be taken seriously. Some people don't tolerate caffeine very well. It can increase heart rate, raise blood pressure, and make some feel jittery. Caffeine is also a diuretic, so one should make sure to stay well hydrated when taking caffeine. A cup of coffee has about 100 mg of caffeine, whereas caffeine tablets, like Nodoze, have 200 mg. Research has shown that between 200 and 300 mg taken about 30 minutes prior to your workout provides the optimum boost in performance.

- **Beta-Alanine**: A naturally occurring beta amino acid that has been shown to increase the concentration of carnosine in muscles, which works to decrease fatigue and thus enables trainees to do more muscular work. This means that you can train a little harder – a little more weight and/or a couple more reps. Beta-Alanine seems to work best when combined with creatine as is now common in most pre-workout energy formulas. A dose of 3 – 4 grams per day seems to work best.

Gaining Weight

With the rate of obesity going through the roof, we often discount the fact that there are many people out there who want or need to gain weight and have trouble doing so. You might not believe it, but it may actually be more difficult for a naturally thin person to gain weight than it is for a naturally heavy person to lose it. I don't know how many thin guys I've met over the years who want to be bigger, but have a hard time putting on weight, even when they lift weights and eat more. I must admit that I have no concept of not being able to gain weight. There's never been a time in my life when I had trouble gaining weight. I realize it must be frustrating for people to eat a lot and still not be able to gain weight. I envy them, in a way. It would be heaven to be able to eat anything I want and not worry about putting on all those extra pounds.

People who have trouble gaining weight have fast metabolisms. They tend to fidget and move around a lot. In short, their bodies are much more efficient at burning calories. Obviously, someone having trouble gaining weight will have to take in more, many more, calories, in order to overcome their speedy metabolisms. I believe the key to gaining weight is consistency in eating. You must keep the calories coming throughout the day and not be too picky about what you eat. The first priority is meeting a daily calorie total. The next priority is to eat mostly high-quality food, like meat, eggs, vegetables, fruits, grains, and milk products.

No matter what you eat, it's crucial that you create a surplus of between 500 and 1,000 calories above maintenance. Those trying to lose weight must create a caloric deficit, but those individuals are walking a very thin line. They don't want to cut calories too much, since that will slow metabolism and likely eat valuable muscle. And, cutting calories too low becomes unhealthy due to the fact we need a certain amount of food in order to get the nutrients our body needs. Eating to gain weight supplies more nutrients, but one must be somewhat careful, still, not to binge on unhealthy foods, like simple sugars and trans fats. These foods are not healthy for anyone and should be kept to a minimum, even for those trying to eat everything in sight.

To help create a caloric surplus, one should limit their activity as much as feasible. Too much movement is part of the problem. All movement burns calories, and these calories will need to be replaced. Obviously, all high-energy activities – like running and other similar sports – should be curtailed. It's hard for me to tell people to exercise less, especially when I've been harping on the need to exercise more. Intentionally trying to gain weight is an exceptional case, however. Instead of doing three cardio sessions a week, reduce that to two sessions, and reduce the time to no more than 20 minutes at a time. Spend most of your energy on high-intensity weight training, keeping your lifting sessions brief but intense. Lift three or four days a week concentrating on compound movements that hit the major muscle groups. Each workout should last no more than an hour. Hit the weights hard, eat plenty of good food, and get plenty of rest.

Gaining Muscle

You can't underestimate the importance of good nutrition when trying to add new muscle. Sound nutrition is second only to intense training, which is necessary to stimulate muscular hypertrophy. Gaining weight is one thing; gaining lean muscle is quite another. When people claim that they've gained a certain amount of muscle, what they really mean, in most cases, is that they've gained some muscle and some fat, and too often, mostly fat. While it is possible to gain muscle without increasing calories above maintenance, it's rare, especially for experienced lifters. People claim to have lost fat and gained muscle at the same time. Once again, this is possible but highly unlikely, except for those who are new to working out. So, to gain muscle, most people have to be in a caloric surplus over an extended span of time. New muscle tissue has to come from somewhere. Your body requires additional energy to build new muscle, including the energy needed to fuel the intense workouts required to stimulate new muscle growth and the additional energy to maintain it after it has been built.

Because it's so difficult to add muscle without taking in more calories, one must be careful not to gain too much bodyfat during the process. Bulking up used to be common, and still is to some extent. This is where guys would eat vast amounts of food while training hard in the gym, in the hope that all those calories would spur muscle growth to the highest degree possible. Bulking up certainly works, as many guys are able to gain a lot of weight and strength to go along with it. The problem is that at least as much of the weight gained is fat as it is muscle. Then, when guys drop their calories in an attempt to "cut" or rid themselves of bodyfat, they end up losing most, if not all, of the muscle they worked so hard to gain. The problem with having to lose a lot of fat is that, inevitably, some muscle is lost during the dieting process. To help avoid this problem – whether trying to gain or lose weight – it's critical that you not alter your caloric intake too drastically. If you add too many calories, you increase the risk of gaining fat, and if you cut calories too much, you increase the likelihood of losing muscle.

Based on all the research I've seen, it's hard to get around the fact that in order to gain muscle, you must be in a caloric surplus. But, how much of a surplus? Another way to look at it is to ask how many calories are needed to build a pound of muscle? We know that a pound of fat contains 3,500 calories, but is this the same for a pound of muscle? This is a very difficult question to answer precisely, since the process of adding muscle varies among individuals. It's obvious, for example, that some people store fat more easily than others, while some are able to pack on muscle faster than others. Building muscle is a complicated process. Providing the physical stimulus via intense training is the first step. Assuming that that has occurred, the body assembles proteins to gradually increase the size of individual muscle fibers. This process involves a myriad of chemical processes, all of which require energy.

It can, to some extent. Stored bodyfat is available to supply us energy when needed. This explains how some people, especially those new to weight training, can lose fat and gain muscle at the same time. While stored fat can be utilized for needed energy, it cannot convert to protein, and additional protein is necessary to add muscle. The main reason our stored fat is not sufficient to fully fuel the muscle-building process is this: Our bodies, through evolution, have been programmed to store extra calories as fat, not muscle. Think of it like this: Once again, it's all about energy and the conservation of energy. It takes much less energy for the body to store a pound of fat than to build a pound of muscle. Muscle requires energy to stimulate its growth, then to fuel the building process, and finally additional energy to maintain it. This process really brings home the reason why it's so difficult to gain muscle but so easy to gain fat.

So, to get back to the question of how many additional calories we need to build a pound of muscle. I recommend that you eat as much as you can without gaining too much fat. Obviously, ectomorphs can get away with eating more and basically anything they want without gaining much weight. The problem for them is not being able to eat enough. Ectomorphs may be able to add anywhere from 500 to 1,000 additional calories above maintenance in order to build muscle. Endomorphs, on the other hand, must be very careful, due to the fact that they gain fat easily. Thus, those of this body type should start by adding only 200 to 300 additional calories a day above maintenance. The more you can eat the better, as more food means more energy and nutrients. This means that you will need to closely monitor your waistline and cut back on calories, if necessary.

Most people assume that additional calories need to come primarily from protein. True, additional protein is important, but it does not need to be taken to such extreme levels as many bodybuilders do. Obviously, you do need more protein to build new muscle, but you need more of everything, including fat, carbs, and micronutrients. The main thing you need when attempting to add muscle are calories. Your total caloric intake is much more important than the amount of protein, or any of the other macronutrients, in the muscle-building process. So, in short, the number of additional calories you need above maintenance to gain a pound of muscle remains undetermined. It's safe to say, though, that one needs about as many additional calories as it takes to add a pound of fat.

How I Gained 10 Pounds of Muscle in 6 Months (at age 50)

Keep in mind that adding new muscle becomes increasingly more difficult the longer you work out. Your muscles adapt to all the stressors placed on them via your workouts and over the years become increasingly resistant to new growth. And the aging process only compounds this. As men get into their 40s, testosterone and growth hormone begin to decline gradually. Both hard gainers and those over 40 can gain muscle, but you need a plan and you need to be persistent and consistent. Here's the plan I used to gain 10 pounds of muscle in 6 months. I went from 220 to 230 pounds without gaining any fat.

- I increased my daily caloric intake slightly above maintenance. For me, that meant going from 2,400 calories a day to around 2,600 a day. The muscle you are trying to add has to come from somewhere; it takes additional energy to build it. These additional calories amounted to approximately 15 grams of protein, 15 grams of carbs, and 9 grams of fat.

- I worked out 4 days a week following the training program described in Chapter 6. I also employed the high-intensity techniques I described. Keep in mind that it's hard training that creates the stimulus to build muscle. Without that, the best nutrition in the world won't make much difference.

- I cut back on cardio from 150 minutes a week to 80 minutes a week, and this was divided into four 20-minute sessions per week. Cardio is very beneficial for conditioning your cardiovascular system, but too much uses energy that could be used for building muscle, and it interferes with hypertrophy because you're asking your muscles to adapt to two different types of training. My cardio sessions were primarily steady-state (same pace throughout) and employed the elliptical and/or treadmill walking at 4 mph on a 3-5 percent incline.

- Supplements: Creatine monohydrate – 5 grams a day. Beta Alanine – 3 grams daily. On my workout days I used a pre-workout formula that contained these, and other, ingredients, like caffeine, for example. This is the only caffeine I used.

- I tried to sleep 7-8 hours a night and even catch a brief power-nap during my lunch break at work. I can't stress enough the importance of trying to simplify your life. Stress in an unavoidable part of life, but don't go out of your way to bring more drama into your life. Too much stress and worry can really hamper your workouts.

Perspective

The whole subject of nutrition can be very confusing. I hope that I haven't added to your confusion. After all is said and done, here are some simple truths to remember.

- Calories matter. The only way to lose fat is to create a caloric deficit over time.
- What we eat is not as important as how much we eat.
- The proportion of carbs, protein, and fat doesn't matter as much as total calories when trying to lose or gain weight.
- Protein is important, especially for building muscle, but mega amounts of protein are not necessary. Divide your bodyweight in half. That's approximately how many grams of protein you need per day. Those seeking to gain muscle can take .7 to .8 grams per pound of bodyweight.
- We already have a pretty good idea which foods are good for us and which ones aren't so good. We can't go wrong by eating more fresh fruits, vegetables, whole grains, legumes, lean dairy, and lean meats. We would probably be better off eating less red meat, sugar-laden foods, and processed foods in general.
- We are what we eat, but food has the potential to bring us much pleasure. So there is always a fine line between always eating what is good for us and indulging one's taste buds and cravings through food. I believe that we can eat much of what we want, within reason, and still be fit and healthy.

11. THE DARK SIDE of EXERCISE

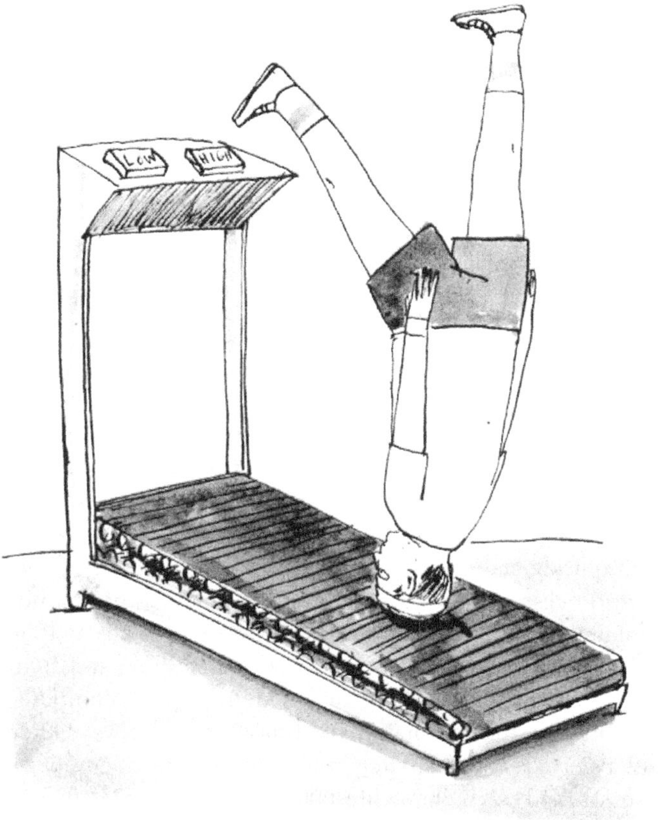

Take care of your body. It's the only place you have to live.
– Jim Rohn

Although I advocate a bodybuilding approach to achieving one's fitness goals, I am not encouraging everyone to become competitive bodybuilders or to get so caught up in your training and your appearance that you lose sight of what's really important, like your health and your relationships. Those wanting to achieve high levels of fitness, must set lofty goals in order to maximize their potential. Accomplishing these goals requires deep and sustained passion and commitment. However, there's a fine line between passion and fanaticism – commitment and compulsiveness. Professional athletes can afford to devote more time to training, since they are getting paid for what they do. Common trainees have other responsibilities and commitments, like work, family, and social life. Life is about tradeoffs. People must be able to balance their fitness aspirations with all their other commitments. Those who devote too much attention to fitness inevitably must sacrifice in other areas of their life. It's when those sacrifices keep you from growing, or even functioning, in other important areas, that your fitness pursuits may become unhealthy.

I have been involved in bodybuilding for nearly 30 years. I have owned a gym and competed in bodybuilding contests. I have spent a lot of time with hardcore bodybuilders and other fitness fanatics. Believe me, some people who get into bodybuilding and other physical pursuits, become obsessed with it, to the point that they devote an inordinate amount of time and resources to it, at the expense of developing other important aspects of their lives. One's life can quickly get out of balance. In this respect, physical endeavors, like bodybuilding, can become like an addiction, and, when taken to the extreme, can rob you of the things you hold dearest.

I must admit that I enjoy the attention I get because of my physique. Compliments from others motivate me and makes all the hard work worthwhile. And the idea that I can look good enough to pose on a stage in less than my underwear is a sublime feeling. Competitive bodybuilding, however, can quickly take over your life, as one must devote so much time, effort, and resources to contest preparation. It's hard to have a normal life and be absolutely committed to your preparation. It's extremely tough on relationships. Weeks of strict dieting leaves one irritable and hard to live with, which further strains relationships. Many of the competitors take anabolic steroids, so the temptation to follow suit is always there. Over time, anabolic steroids can absolutely ruin your health, which nullifies many of the plusses of the bodybuilding lifestyle.

Maybe surprisingly, many bodybuilders – at least the competitive ones – aren't that concerned with their health. While competitors look healthy with their tanned, bulging muscles under the stage lights, bodybuilders at the time of competition are anything but healthy. They are extremely depleted due to weeks of strict dieting. They've deprived themselves of water and even taken diuretics to further rid themselves of water under the skin. It's common to see bodybuilders have to pull out of a competition due to severe cramping brought on by dehydration. Some have even died from it. And let's not forget the damage that anabolic steroids may be doing to their internal organs. While competitive bodybuilders look superhuman on the outside, their muscles hide problems on the inside.

Bodybuilders are good examples of obsessed trainees, but they aren't the only ones, not by a long shot. Extreme endurance athletes may be even worse. I'm referring primarily to those who compete in marathons and triathlons. A marathon is 26.2 miles. Why someone would want to run this far nonstop is a mystery to me, but it's a goal for many. The amount of weekly running required to train for a marathon is extreme, to say the least. It's not uncommon for people training for a marathon to log a 100 miles a week. This is overtaining to the max, not to mention all the wear and tear on the body. What's worse, ultra-marathons – races of 60 and up to 100 miles – are becoming more popular. This is insanity! The pinnacle of endurance competitions is unquestionably the Ironman triathlon, first held in Hawaii. This grueling race consists of triathlons, consisting of a mere 2.4-mile swim, a 112-mile bike ride, and then to top it off, a full marathon. People want to do it just to say that they've done it. And I must admit, it is quite an accomplishment to simply complete an event as challenging as this, let alone win one. My concern, though, is the inordinate amount of time and effort that must be devoted to training for not only one but three different events, with each one being a feat in itself.

One should always be mindful that exercise is stress upon the body, which accumulates along with all other stressors in our lives. This might sound contradictory, since we often hear that exercise is a great stress reliever. What actually occurs when we exercise is that the brain releases powerful chemicals called endorphins in response to the perceived stress – increased heart rate, physical exertion, lactic acid buildup from muscle contractions. So, exercise is stress that is actually beneficial, so long as it's not carried on for too long. Research has shown that most people derive the maximum good-feeling effect from endorphins with only about 20-30 minutes of exercise daily. This seems to vary widely among individuals and may explain why some people literally become addicted to exercise while others hate it with a passion. The bottom line is that stress, all sorts of stress, is cumulative and therefore must be managed or it will produce a deleterious effect on one's health.

One might think that being addicted to exercise would be a good thing, but it's not. The diagnosed condition, called activity anorexia, for example, causes poor, not good, health. Activity anorexia is a vicious cycle where a drastic decrease in eating leads to progressively more exercise, which leads to even less eating. In experiments done on rats, a reduction in food actually causes rats to spend more time, not less, on the running wheel. Some rats continue to run more than others, even when food is increased. Those rats showed signs of ill health and would have died, if left to continue their destructive behavior. Another condition, known as the binge/purge syndrome, people binge on food and then engage in insane amounts of exercise in an attempt to burn off what they consumed. This practice is unhealthy, since both overeating and then over-exercising are both counterproductive.

Our culture places a great premium on physical appearance, especially among women. Women are bombarded with images of how attractive women are supposed to look, and they are nearly always thin. Female models and movie stars are notorious for being ultra-thin to the point of being frail and unhealthy. Many experts feel that the added pressure from the media to be thin has contributed to a rise in anorexia nervosa among women, and increasingly among men as well. Those with this condition see themselves as being fat, although they are thin. This distorted body image leads one to over-exercise, in addition to under-eating, in an effort to become thinner. Tragically, between 5 and 20 percent of those with the condition will die. On the opposite end of the body self-image scale lies body dysmorphic disorder, a condition where people see a distorted image of their body. Many men with this condition see themselves as being smaller than they really are. Even brawny, muscular men with this condition never think that they are big or muscular enough, and thus search for ways to get bigger. This leads men to spend hours training in the gym and taking all sorts of dietary supplements to help them gain more muscle. It also compels many to take anabolic steroids, which can be harmful if taken in high doses or taken for over an extended period of time.

Many well-intentioned people who begin exercise programs overdo it and end up injuring themselves. Injuries are the bane of exercise, since they keep people from improving their fitness. Even experienced trainees incur injuries, some of which become chronic while others sideline trainees for weeks or months at a time. There's a very fine line between pushing past your current limits and pushing too hard or too fast. As I mentioned before, exercise is stress, and stress must be managed. It's ironic that the one activity that can do your body the most good – regular intense exercise – also has the potential to do serious harm. To avoid injuries, I recommend that trainees pay attention to the following training protocols:

- Learn how to do exercises correctly and safely. Beginners might consider working with a personal trainer until your confident to go at it alone.
- Stay away from heavy single repetitions. A maximum attempt increases the chances of a muscle or tendon tear.
- Be careful when doing high-impact, or explosive, movements, like plyometrics, for example. This type of exercise has its place (mainly for trained athletes), but, once again, increases the chances of injury.
- Know your limitations. After training for a while, you begin to learn which exercises produce pain (and not the good kind, either). Avoid exercises that cause you pain, or at least keep the weight down. I've been training for over 30 years, and there are certain exercises that I avoid.

Perspective

My advice for anyone pursuing physical perfection is to strive for balance in your life. Obviously, you must be committed to hard work and perseverance, but there's a fine line between commitment – which is a generally a good thing – and fanaticism – which is almost always a bad thing. Looking good and being fit and healthy are important ends in themselves, but not at the expense of other equally or more important ends, like family, friends, and relationships. The things that will bring you the most happiness in life are the times you spend with others. Make those times count. Gaining the perspective from seeing the big picture will help you achieve the proper balance.

12. Mind / MUSCLE

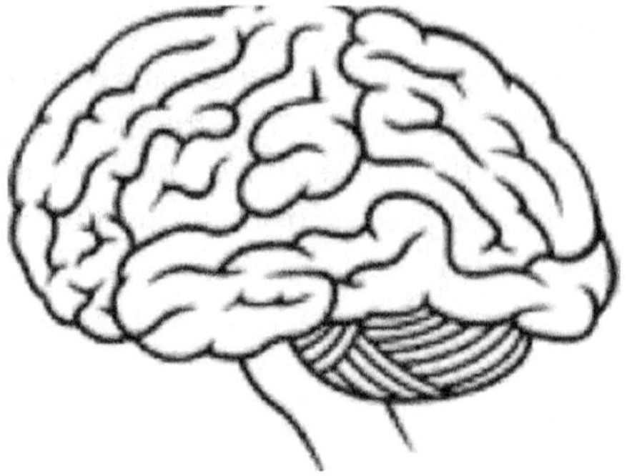

This needs exercise, too!

Dispositions of the mind, like limbs of the body, acquire strength by exercise. – Thomas Jefferson

With all the focus on the physical aspects of fitness, it's easy to neglect the mental side of things. I contend that the mental aspects are at least as, if not more, important than the physical. The meaning of life is to find purpose in life. Taking care of our bodies and being healthy should be one important purpose for us. And, as I've argued throughout this book, people simply cannot maximize their fitness potential without simultaneously developing one's mental potential. There is ample evidence now showing that engaging in physical exercise enhances our mental capabilities. I argue that the reverse is also true.

Maximizing fitness may require us to change how we think. There's the notion, for example, that people should do whatever they can to avoid physical labor. This way of thinking comes from the time when people had to perform a lot of work to get by and looked for ways to make their lives easier. At the same time, people think it's smart to avoid work, as if they take pride in showing off their ingenuity. It's amazing how creative and resourceful people can be when they want to avoid hard, physical labor, or mental labor, for that matter. Inactivity is killing us. We should be looking for ways to move and work more, not less. And I'm not just talking about your workouts. Working out on a regular basis is a given, an integral part of your life. I'm referring to your lifestyle.

One way to change your life for the better is to develop good habits. Your willpower can be strong, but good habits can help keep you on the right path when your willpower falters from time to time.

Productive Daily Habits

Good habits are as addictive as bad habits, and a lot more rewarding.
– Author Unknown

- **Exercise every day and strenuously four days a week:** Regular exercise is the basis for fitness and sound health. Exercise also helps control your weight, relieves stress, and elevates mood.
- **Read something:** Reading is the best thing you can do to build your mental power and to gain knowledge. You should read all you can about fitness, nutrition, and everything else.
- **Practice the Golden Rule:** This is a very simple yet effective philosophy of life: "Do unto others as you would have them do unto you." Just think how much better the world would be if everyone followed this one simple rule.
- **Challenge your brain:** We know that physical exercise actually helps the brain perform better. The reverse may also be true. Stimulating the brain can enhance fitness. The body, including your muscles, is a vast neural network, which is controlled by the brain. Enhancing the brain, then, contributes to faster movement of neural signaling within this complex network. As mentioned previously, reading is an excellent way to stimulate the brain and accumulate knowledge. Greater knowledge leads to better training and diet. Engaging in critical thinking enables people to make better decisions regarding their fitness program. Other ways of enhancing our brain include doing crosswords and other puzzles, playing board games and cards, learning a foreign language or how to play a musical instrument.
- **Visualize your goals and intentions:** There's a wise old saying that "the best way to predict the future is to create it." Some people contend that our thoughts can influence the physical world. If this is true, then it makes a strong case for promoting positive thinking while avoiding negative thoughts. A major part of positive thinking is to see, as clearly as possible in your mind, exactly what you want to accomplish. I believe that visualizing the future we want – our goals and intentions – helps us to make them real. Try visualizing

exactly how you want your body to look and work at realizing it. I even visualize my workouts. I rehearse them in my mind – the exercises, sets, and reps – before I get to the gym. In that sense, I've already done the workout. Visualizing my workouts this way helps me to focus more clearly on the exercises while I'm actually doing them.

- **Make a to-do list**: Anyone interested in being more productive and efficient needs a daily to-do list. I find that a list does the following: 1) It keeps me focused on what I need to get done; 2) It helps me prioritize things; and 3) Gives me a sense of accomplishment when I'm able to check things off.
- **Be on time:** Promptness is an important character trait. It demonstrates dependability. Also, doing things daily at regular times instills routine and a sense of predictability. Call me boring, but I find great comfort in following a daily routine.
- **Smile more often:** Nothing is more pleasing than to be greeted by someone with a bright smile, and I believe that smiles are contagious. Others will respond to you more favorably if you smile more often. The easiest way to improve the world is through more smiles.
- **Eat healthy:** In the promotion of health and fitness, good nutrition ranks right up there with exercise. All of us can make better choices about what we eat without being too radical. Like most things, moderation is the key.
- **Do something good for someone else:** I firmly believe in the practice of paying it forward, or doing something kind for someone else without expecting anything in return. In fact, the true test of character is what you do when no one is watching – or what you do when you know you will not get credit for it. And, if you believe in karma, then doing good for others always comes back to you eventually.
- **Get enough sleep:** Sleep plays a vital role in all aspects of our lives, not just in health and fitness. Sleep is when we recover and refresh. Lack of adequate sleep leaves the body in a weakened condition, which hinders normal functioning. Most days I even try to get in a short nap.
- **Practice self-reflection and critical thinking**: You should reflect on your life regularly as a means of self-assessment. Be honest with yourself and always seek to improve. You should also think critically about your own thinking and question everything, including your own thinking and assumptions. Above all, you should get in the habit of thinking for yourself.

Go With the Flow

Another good habit is the cultivation of flow. Flow is what psychologists refer to as the state of mind when one is immersed in an activity that requires concentration and focus. Another way of describing flow is the complete absorption in what one is doing. Some common terms associated with flow include in the zone, in the moment, centered, in the groove, or in tune. Picture someone so engrossed in an activity that they lose touch with their surroundings. You might wonder whether this is a good state to be in. It is. Being in flow energizes and brings joy to the participant, which contributes to the successful completion of complex tasks.

Fortunately, flow can be applied to exercise. In fact, you need flow to get the most out of your workouts. Training at a high level of intensity requires total concentration. Imagine doing a set of heavy squats, where you are shooting for 10 reps. You know that 10 reps are going to be tough, so much so that you have someone spot you, just in case you need a little help on the final rep. You begin by focusing on the difficult task at hand. You get under the bar, lift it off the supports, and step back. You get your feet set and take a deep breath. Now you must concentrate on nothing but moving the weight. You block out your surroundings. You fight through the pain as you complete rep after rep. You have your spotter call out the reps because you are too focused on the lift to keep an accurate count. You reach your goal of 10, and a euphoric-like feeling of accomplishment surges through you as you rack the bar. Your surroundings become palpable to you again. You loosen your belt and try your best to catch your breath. You rest for a couple of minutes and do it all over again.

This is what my workouts are like – periods of intense concentration interspersed with brief periods of rest. The rest periods are as important for the recovery of mental, as well as, physical exercise. The ability to focus all of one's attention on a singular task is paramount to performing physically at one's best. It's no wonder that most people avoid hard work. Intense exercise is very demanding, even painful. Our natural inclination is to avoid pain and conserve energy. Engaging in arduous, painful tasks requires the utmost determination, which depends on one being able to focus intently on that single task. This ability must be developed over time. As you become more acclimated to exercise, you learn to push yourself a little harder. Then, reaching your short-term goals propels you to train even harder. Here are a few suggestions for developing flow in regard to exercise:

- Set clear, realistic, and short-term goals. Doing this will set you up for progress, and progress will motivate you to continue and to push yourself further. The longer you train, the better you become at focusing.

- If you are new to working out, think about getting a personal trainer, at least until you have enough experience to feel confident doing all the exercises. The better you become at doing an exercise, the more you are able to focus your full attention on challenging your muscles, instead of on your form. A good trainer can push and motivate you and then teach you how to motivate yourself.
- Work out with someone. Training partners can be a major motivator. You always have a spotter – someone pushing you – and you have to try and outdo your partner. There's nothing like a little competition to motivate people.
- Practice visualization. Rehearse your workouts, even particular exercises, before you do them, as this mental coaching sets the stage for you to experience flow.
- Practice, practice, practice: Perhaps the best way to develop flow is to intentionally think about it; make it happen. This gets to the heart of mind over matter, or in this case mind over muscle. Concentrate only on the task at hand while trying your best to block out the rest of the world.

The Fitness Lifestyle

Success is the sum of small efforts, repeated day in and day out.
– R. Collier

People often ask me why I exercise so much. I usually respond by asking them why they exercise so little. For me, exercising is in the same category as sleeping and eating. It's essential. It's just something I do every day, and it's just as important to me as all the other things I do on a daily basis. I make exercise a high priority in my life. When it's time for my workout, I work out. If it's time for my walk and it's raining, I take my umbrella. If it's -10F outside, dress appropriately. There really are no excuses. You just do it.

Regular, structured workouts are only part of the fitness equation, albeit an important one. The fitness lifestyle also entails all the other exercise you do in addition to your regular workouts. A good example is taking the stairs instead of the elevator, and doing so on a regular basis. If you have an office job, you can spend your break walking. The trick to developing these types of behaviors is to gradually make them habits. To do so requires you to consciously think about your behaviors and to make appropriate choices. And when you are presented with a choice, always choose the option that requires you to move more or work harder. Most people do the opposite. They look for the easiest way to get something done or the shortest distance between two points. We must overcome our inclinations to avoid work by seeking ways to work more. Here are some examples of choosing to work more instead of less:

- Always take the stairs instead of the elevator or escalator.
- Consciously take more steps during the day. This means when you have to walk somewhere, take the longer route. Wearing a pedometer is a good way to keep up with your total number of steps.
- Park a longer distance from where you are going, like at work or the mall. There's always plenty of parking spaces at the back of the lot. You're also less likely to get your car dinged out there.
- When grocery shopping, go up and down every aisle and all around the perimeter of the store, even if you don't need anything in that particular aisle. The idea here, once again, is to get into the habit of walking more. And you'll burn more calories since you are pushing a cart. I even load the heavy items first as to get the benefit of pushing more weight for a longer period of time. Just be careful not to fill your cart with unhealthy and high-calorie foods. They will call out to you. I know that at some stores the baggers still take your cart out and load your car for you. Do this yourself, unless you are in a wheelchair or something.
- When shopping at the mall make sure you complete a couple of laps walking around the entire mall.
- Unless you have an acre of yard, mow your lawn with a push mower. This is one of the best workouts around – push/pull resistance, stretching, and plenty of cardio.

In the end fitness is about little things, and the little things add up over time to make significant differences.

13. MY 12-WEEK FITNESS CHALLENGE

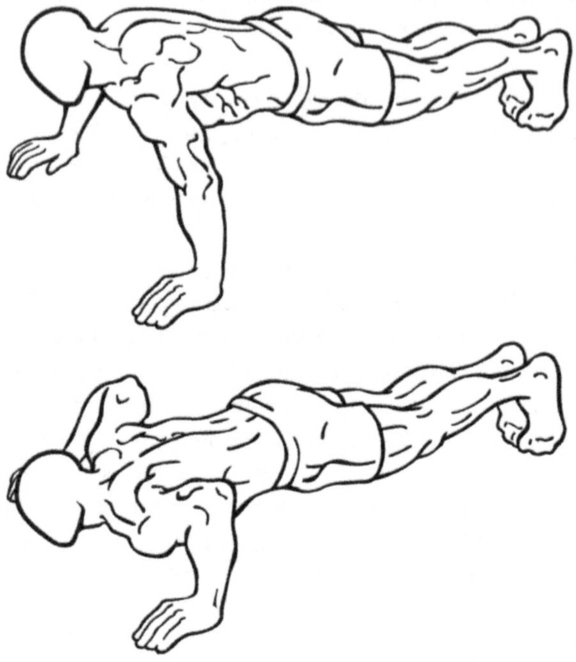

The following plan is designed to get you focused on a few key exercises and chart your improvement over a period of time. While I emphasize life-long fitness behaviors, people new, or returning to regular exercise, respond better to a defined time constraint – in this case, 12 weeks. I encourage you to utilize the charts included with this plan to chart your progress. Being able to record improvements will help to motivate you.

Exercises

Level I: By level I, I mean that these exercises can be performed, at least minimally, by most people and require little, if any additional equipment.

Mile Run/Walk: This is arguably the best test of one's cardiovascular fitness. Don't worry if you can't run a mile. Start out be walking and running, with improvement in time as your goal.

Pushups: Pushups are a good test of upper-body strength, and you can do them virtually anywhere without any additional equipment.

Situps: Situps are still a good test of abdominal muscle (core) strength and endurance, no matter what people say. And, like pushups, you can do them almost anywhere. You should secure your feet, or have someone hold them. While lying on your back, bend your knees to where they are pointing straight up. With your hands behind your head, bring your upper body up to where you can touch your elbows to your knees.

Level II: Level II exercises are more difficult and require some special equipment.

Pullups: Often called chin-ups, pullups test your pulling strength. You must begin with your arms fully extended while gripping the bar and feet off the floor. 1 rep consists of pulling yourself from this position up until your chin is slightly above the bar and then returning to the stating position before beginning another rep. Don't worry about how you grasp the bar – palms facing you or facing away. You might want to try both grips, as the palms facing in works the biceps a little more than palms facing out. Pull-ups are difficult because pulling your entire bodyweight against gravity is something that we rarely do.

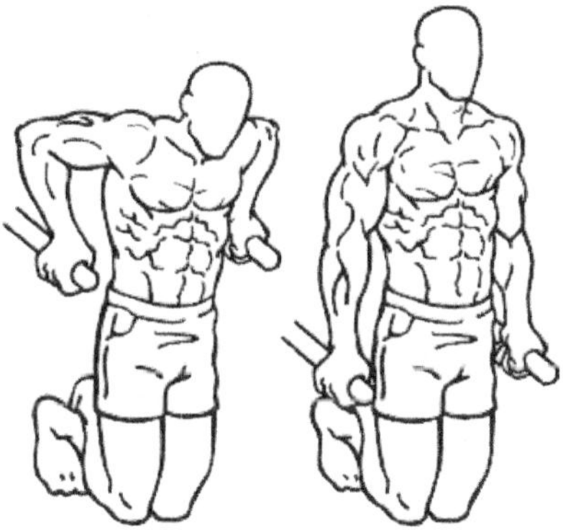

Dips: Dips are performed by grasping parallel bars with arms fully extended, lowering your body between the bars until your upper arms are parallel with the bars, and then pushing yourself back to the starting point (arms extended). In my opinion, the dip is the best all-around upper-body exercise in the book, as it challenges the pecs, triceps, and delts almost equally. Dips are very challenging, since you are moving your entire bodyweight through space. Few women can do a correct dip, since most women lack the required upper body strength. Heck, most men can't do a correct dip.

Max Bench Press: The bench press is a good test of upper-body strength and power. A good goal is to bench more than your bodyweight. Caution: Always use a spotter when going for your max on the bench. I have gotten a loaded bar stuck on my chest before, and it's not a pleasant experience.

Bench Press x Bodyweight: This is a difficult test and a real challenge for people who have been lifting for a while and have built up some good strength and endurance. Keep in mind that many people can't even bench press their bodyweight one time.

Level III: Level III exercise is distinguished by being extremely demanding and requiring practice to perform correctly.

Deadlift Max: The deadlift is, arguably, the most demanding exercise, since it works so many muscles. Before attempting your max, practice the lift until you have developed impeccable form. Sloppy form on this lift will lead to injury. I often use the diamond, or trap, bar, which allows you to grip the bar on the sides of your body instead of in the front. This keeps the bar closer to your center of gravity, which allows for greater leg drive and reduces slightly the stress placed on the lower back. I recommend wearing a lifting belt while doing deadlifts to help support your lower back and core. I also use straps for my heaviest sets to help with my grip.

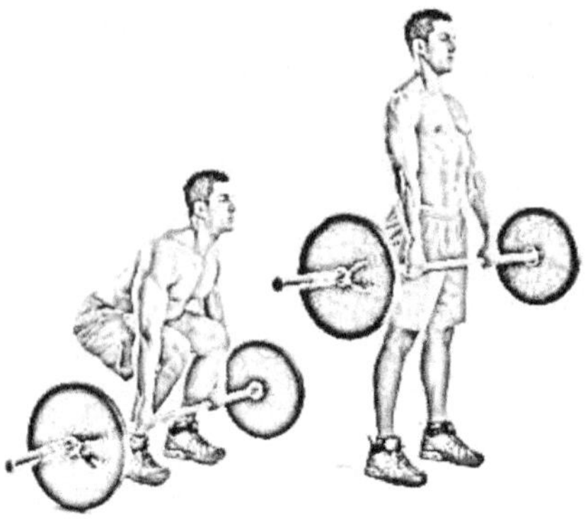

Deadlift x Bodyweight: Like the bench press, you should be able to deadlift your bodyweight. After training for a while, a good goal would be to increase your total number of reps using your bodyweight. This lift is so demanding, that if you can do 10 reps, or more, with your body weight, you will be breathing like you've just run a 100-yard dash. Do several sets like this, and you have one of the best cardio (and resistance) workouts ever. Talk about revving your metabolism! You can't beat it.

Setting Realistic Goals

The first thing to do is test yourself on each of these measures and record your results. Keep in mind that these are simply measures of fitness. They are something that fit people can do. However, they don't necessarily have to be part of your workout schedule. Due to the transfer principle, you can improve in one exercise by doing a related exercise. At the same time, though, these are basic exercises, and I recommend that you do them. If you are a beginner, you can base your whole workout around these basic exercises. If you are more advanced, you can incorporate them into your routine. I still do each of these exercises regularly.

In setting goals, it's important to know what outcomes might and might not be realistic. If you can't do a pushup, for example, a good goal would be to be able to do one. Once you can do one, set your sights on doing two, and so forth. Adding one pushup a week would be a reasonable goal. If you are below average in the number of reps or weight you can do, then a reasonable goal for the 12-week challenge may be to bring yourself up to average. Keep in mind that for exercises like the bench press, your weight is a factor. You can't compare your max to that of people who weigh a lot more than you do. Similarly, bodyweight comes into play on pullups and dips, since the more you weight, the harder it will be to pull or push yourself up. Simply losing weight (hopefully fat) will help you perform better on these exercises. The most important thing is to make some improvement, no matter how small. Once again, here are the averages for these exercises:

Average and Great Performance on Basic Exercises

Exercise	Female		Male	
	Average	Great	Average	Great
Mile Run/Walk	11 min.	7.5 min.	10 min.	6 min.
Pushups (1 minute)	20*	10	30	50
Situps (1 minute)	35	55	45	70
Pullups	<1	4	3	12
Bench Press Max	90	150	150	300
Bench Press, Reps x Bodyweight	<1	3	1	10
Deadlift Max	135	195	200	350
Deadlift, Reps x Bodyweight	1	5	3	11

*Number of "girl" pushups.

Performance Goals for the 12-Week Challenge

Exercise	Current Level	Goal (12 Week)
Mile Run/Walk		
Pushups (1 minute)		
Situps (1 minute)		
Pullups		
Bench Press Max		
Bench Press x Bodyweight		
Deadlift Max		
Deadlift x Bodyweight		

Workout Schedule

I'm not going to write one single workout for everyone to follow. I have provided you with my own workout, but everyone is different and at different points in their development. The type of workout you follow should be based primarily on your goals and your level of training experience. Beginners, for example, don't require a complicated workout in order to make gains. A few exercises performed a few times a week will do the trick. Someone who is more advanced will need a more complicated workout, like mine, for example. What I want is for people to start thinking critically about their training, and thus use a number of sources in developing an individual training program.

The idea behind the 12-week challenge is to take your fitness to the next level, no matter where you are right now. Ideally, I recommend engaging in some sort of exercise on a daily basis, mainly to instill good habits. Your daily exercise doesn't have to be an intense workout; it can be a leisurely walk, gardening, or housework. Below are two workout schedules, based on whether you are trying to lose or gain weight.

The workouts are coded as followed: 1=intense resistance training; 2=moderate to intense cardio (i.e. jogging); 3=light cardio (i.e. walking).

Weekly Training Schedule for Weight Loss						
M	T	W	TH	F	SAT	SUN
1, 3	2	1, 3	2	1, 3	2	3
Weekly Training Schedule for Weight Gain						
M	T	W	TH	F	SAT	SUN
1	1	2	1	3	1	3

Note the differences in the two workouts. Basically, if you are trying to lose weight, you need to move more and thus burn more calories, and when trying to gain weight, move less and conserve calories. Therefore, the weight loss plan calls for more moderate-to-intense cardio and more light cardio, while the weight gain plan calls for less cardio and more intense resistance work. I have included only one-week examples for each plan. Over the course of 12 weeks, the schedule doesn't change, but the workouts get more intense and/or longer. Each week you must try to increase what you did the previous week. As stated previously, your starting point depends on your current level of fitness. Here are rough examples of what these three workouts might look like:

1 – Intense Resistance Workout: A full-body workout consisting of several sets of exercises that impact the major muscle groups, such as squats, deadlifts, bench presses, and pullups, among others. This workout should last about 45 minutes to an hour at most. Do 2 to 3 sets of 8 to 12 reps on each exercise and try to lift a little more weight each workout.

2 – Moderate-to-Intense Cardio: In this workout, you elevate your heart rate for an extended period of time. The best way to accomplish this is by jogging or utilizing a cardio machine. Many like to vary their intensity during the workout by alternating between high- and low-intensity intervals. This workout should last between 30 and 45 minutes. One increases intensity by training faster and/or longer, i.e. doing more work in a given period of time.

3 – Light Cardio: This workout consists of more leisurely activities like walking, for example. Actually, one can engage in any type of cardio activity, just at a slower pace. This means that the activity can be conducted for a longer period of time. This workout can last anywhere from 30 minutes to well over an hour, as in the case of a good hike, for example. There's no need to try and increase the intensity of these workouts, but you could increase the duration and frequency of these workouts without worrying about overtraining.

The tables on the following pages are designed to help you keep track of your progress, both training and diet. Copy or modify them to fit your individualized needs.

Use the tables below (**Performance Measures**) and (**Body Measures**) to keep track of your progress over your 12-week fitness plan.

Week	Performance Measures								
	Mile Run	Push ups	Pull ups	Sit ups	Dips	Max Bench	Bench x BW	Max Dead	Dead x BW
1									
2									
3									
4									
5									
6									
7									
8									
9									
10									
11									
12									

Weeks	**Body Measures**					
	Weight	BMI	Waist	Hips	RHR	BP
1						
2						
3						
4						
5						
6						
7						
8						
9						
10						
11						
12						

Use the following tables (**Daily Training Log** and **Daily Food Log**) to keep track of your daily training and nutrition.

Daily Training Log				
Body Part		**Date**	**Time**	**Total Training Time**
Exercise	**Set**	**Weight**	**Reps**	**Notes**
Body Part				
Body Part				

Daily Food Log				
	Foods	**Time**	**Macronutrients**	**Total Calories**
Meal 1			Carbs	
			Protein	
			Fat	
Meal 2			Carbs	
			Protein	
			Fat	
Meal 3			Carbs	
			Protein	
			Fat	
Meal 4			Carbs	
			Protein	
			Fat	
Meal 5			Carbs	
			Protein	
			Fat	
Snacks			Carbs	
			Protein	
			Fat	
Total			Carbs	
			Protein	
			Fat	

The Fitness Index

I'm repeating the Fitness Index here that I introduced in Chapter 2. Use the table below to score yourself on the measures included in the assessment and calculate your Fitness Index.

Fitness Index			
Measure	**Description**	**Points**	**Score**
Pushups	The number of pushups completed in 1 minute	1 point for each rep completed	
Situps	The number of situps completed in 1 minute	1 point for each rep completed	
Dips	The number of dips completed in 1 minute	1 point for each rep completed	
Pullups	The number of pullups completed in 1 minute	1 point for each rep completed	
Bench Press x Bodyweight	The number of reps completed in 1 minute using one's bodyweight	2 points for each rep completed	
Deadlift x Bodyweight	The number of reps completed in 1 minute using one's bodyweight	2 points for each rep completed	
Subtotal	Scores of above measures added together		
1-Mile Run/Walk	The time it takes to run/walk 1 mile	Total time x 2 and that number subtracted from the subtotal	
Grand Total	Subtotal minus score for 1-mile run/walk		

Rating Scale

<40 = Below Average
41 – 70 = Average
71 – 100 = Good
101 – 140 = Excellent
141 – 180 = Remarkable
181 – 220 = Freakish
221 and above = Superhuman

Keep in mind, also, the modifications for women discussed in Chapter 2.

EPILOGUE

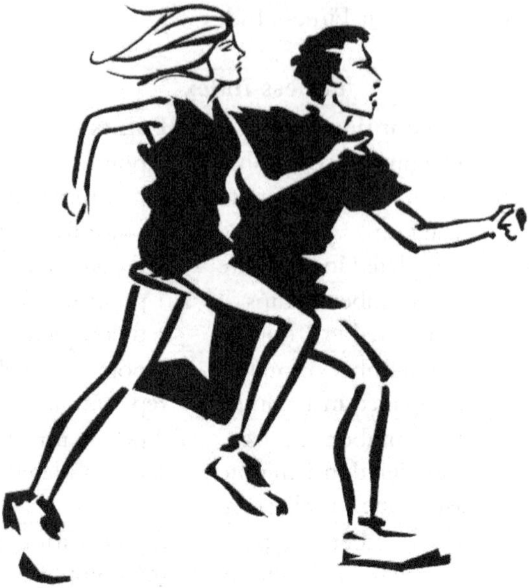

It is health that is real wealth and not pieces of gold and silver.
– Mahatma Gandhi

My goals in writing this book were 1) to help readers explore issues related to the personal enhancement of fitness; 2) to get readers to think more critically about fitness and related issues; and 3) challenge readers to improve their own fitness by adopting a fitness lifestyle. I hope I have accomplished what I set out to do.

I have argued for a modified bodybuilding approach to fitness, which is to say that I believe it to be the most productive and efficient means to achieving and maintaining high levels of fitness. This, however, is by no means the only path to fitness. Much depends on where you are and how far you want to go. If you get nothing else out of this book, remember that some exercise is better than no exercise, and, correspondingly, intense exercise is better than lax exercise, to a point. Too much exercise has negative effects on health.

I have referred to my fitness plan as the Cerebral approach. With "Cerebral," I have tried to emphasize the critical thinking and reasoning powers that must be developed in order for us to reach our physical potential.

Summary

Fitness is an expansive topic, touching on several overlapping disciplines and key concepts. I attempted to weave these concepts into an overarching philosophy of fitness, but while writing the book, I feared that I might have bitten off too much for readers to digest. With most topics, I tried to simplify things as much as possible and still convey important information. In doing this, however, I ran the risk of oversimplifying topics to the point of them being virtually meaningless. In reality, I do believe that the concepts surrounding fitness are pretty simple. Execution, though, is where the difficulty comes in. In keeping with my simplicity theme, here is summary of the most important concepts of fitness:

- We are getting fatter and less fit primarily due to eating too much and exercising too little.
- We have to think more critically about fitness, which means questioning everything related to exercise, nutrition, and health.
- Some exercise is better than no exercise.
- Too much exercise can be counterproductive, since it is stress, and stress is cumulative.
- Forming good habits is the key to fitness, and success in general.
- While there is no bad exercise per se, intense resistance exercise should be your primary focus.
- While important to conditioning and health promotion, cardio exercise is somewhat overrated.
- The Cerebral approach takes the best aspects of bodybuilding and combines it with critical thinking.
- Portion control is the key to fat loss.

Recommendations

I've tried to provide a coherent fitness plan for individuals. Now, I want to offer a few, more sweeping, recommendations for society as a whole. Can we, as a species, reverse the course we are on and become more fit. I believe we can; we must. However, it will require us to rethink what we are currently doing and then change our behaviors. For just as one sets the conditions that are more likely to result in success, we, as a society, can create environments for the population at large that are more likely to encourage the promotion of fitness.

- Obviously, we have to develop good habits in children, as they are more likely to carry them into adulthood. Doing this, however, means placing much more attention on fitness in schools.
- A good starting point for our children is to feed them better while they are at school. Our children need and deserve nutritious foods, and eating healthful foods will help them develop better eating habits. Part of the nutrition problem is getting out the obvious junk foods, like sugar-laden sodas, candy, and chips offered via vending machines. These unhealthy snacks can be replaced with more nutritious ones, like fruit, nuts, and lower-calorie snacks.
- In schools throughout the country we could elevate exercise and nutrition to the level of reading and math. It's that important. The revised three R's could be reading, running, and resistance. How about 50 minutes of physical education every school day. Formal instruction in nutrition at each grade level. More recess time for children to simply play. Well-equipped gyms with exercise equipment, including resistance and cardio machines.
- Everyone should have access to a quality fitness facility. There are gyms everywhere in metropolitan areas but not many in rural areas. Plus, many people can't afford gym membership fees. I'd like to see a well-equipped fitness center in every community and with a sliding payment scale based on one's income. One solution is to put fitness centers in schools, as mentioned above, and open them up to the general public in the evenings and on weekends. Maybe federal or state grants could be made available to communities lacking fitness opportunities. Fitness centers would be a good way for philanthropists to help society, similar to the way Carnegie built libraries throughout the country.
- Communities must be planned and organized in a way that encourages, instead of discourages, fitness. Right now in many communities, especially in dense urban areas, it's virtually impossible to walk anywhere, due to the lack of sidewalks and street overpasses. And to ride a bike in most urban areas is to put your life at risk.
- Cities and towns should invest more in parks and recreation. This includes organizing opportunities for exercise like leagues, races, fun runs/walks, dances, and other events and competitions.
- Workplaces could install exercise equipment/facilities, and as an incentive to exercise, encourage their employees to utilize it during work hours.
- Insurance companies could reward people who engage in fitness and make real improvements in their health by reducing their

premiums.

- Public buildings could be designed as to encourage people to use the stairs instead of the elevator or escalator. The way it is now, it's difficult to find the stairs in many public buildings.
- Women should be encouraged to breastfeed their children, and we should do everything we can to accommodate them doing this in public places.
- More public awareness campaigns promoting fitness could be undertaken. Following is a list of current fitness-promoting public awareness and information campaign websites:

- http://www.letsmove.gov/
- http://www.acsm.org/
- http://www.physicalactivityplan.org/
- http://www.physicalfitness.org/
- http://healthyamericans.org/
- http://www.cdc.gov/healthmarketing/
- http://www.activelifemovement.org/
- http://www.health.gov/PAGuidelines/
- http://www.health.gov/dietaryguidelines/
- http://www.aahperd.org/
- http://www.saferoutesinfo.org/
- http://apps.nccd.cdc.gov/DNPAProg/StateV.asp
- http://www.aafp.org/online/en/home/policy/state/links.html
- http://www.nyshepa.org/about_us.php
- http://www.hopsports.com/
- http://www.nga.org/portal/site/nga/menuitem.b14a675ba7f89cf9e8ebb856a11010a0
- http://www.usda.gov/wps/portal/usda/usdahome
- http://www.hhs.gov/
- http://www.hhs.gov/news/press/2010pres/09/20100914b.html
- http://www.apha.org/
- http://www.rwjf.org/
- http://www.rwjf.org/pr/product.jsp?id=71348
- http://www.rwjf.org/pr/product.jsp?id=71427
- http://www.healthy-america.org/

He who has health, has hope; and he who has hope, has everything. – Thomas Carlyle

Fitness will always be a challenge, especially in our current environment. To make significant progress, we must change our behaviors and develop new habits. I firmly believe that if we don't get a handle on this issue, our collective health, mobility, and lifespan will continue to deteriorate. When I say "we," I'm referring to the entire human race. However, the human race is made up of individuals, and it is up to individuals to take charge of their own health and fitness.

Modern medicine, with its myriad of drugs and high-tech equipment, has given us a false sense of security. We rely too much on drugs to cope with disease and discomfort. Got a cold, take a pill. In a bad mood, take a pill. Can't sleep, take a pill. Need energy, take a pill. You get the idea. We've become overly dependent on modern pharmacology to treat all of our ills. Now we expect magic pills that will make us slim and fit overnight. I am doubtful whether such a magic pill will ever exist. If it does, it may come with side effects that will be more harmful than the ill effects of being obese. No, the best answer is for people to adopt a more healthy lifestyle, one that includes the tenets I have presented in this book. One doesn't need to go to extremes in order to enhance fitness. Small changes add up over time to make significant improvements. The future of humanity is up to us. Your future is up to you. You can be leaner, stronger, and healthier. Are you up to the challenge?

REFERENCES & NOTES

With a topic as broad as fitness and the sub-topics that I addressed, the references I could include could be nearly endless in number. So what I've tried to do with this section is to provide the reader with a good representative sample of the things I have read and that have subsequently informed my writing in each of the chapters. In keeping with the theme of critical thinking, I encourage the reader to read extensively in each of these areas. There is no shortage of information out there for those who look for it.

Chapter 1: What is Fitness?

Exercise in general:

Gallup Poll. (September 19, 2012). Americans exercising slightly more in 2012. Online, www.gallup.com

Kravitz, L. (2011). What motivates people to exercise? *IDEA Fitness Journal*, 8(1): 25-27.

Parker, S. Physical fitness and exercise: The facts. Health Guidance.org.

Benefits of exercise:

Ballantyne, C. (January 2, 2009). Does exercise really make you healthier? *Scientific American*: http://www.scientificamerican.com/article.cfm?id=does-exercise-really-make

Kravitz, L. (2008). Yes, resistance training can reverse the aging process. *IDEA Fitness Journal*, 5(8): 21-23.

Landro, L. (January 5, 2010). The hidden benefits of exercise: Even moderate physical activity can boost the immune system and protect against chronic diseases. *The Wall Street Journal*: http://online.wsj.com/article/SB10001424052748704350304574638331243027174.htm

Maddalozzo, G.F., and Snow, C.M. (2000). High intensity resistance training: Effects on bone in older men and women. *Calcified Tissue*

International, 66: 399-404.

Melov, S., Tarnopolsky, M., Beckman, K., & Hubbard, A. (2007). Resistance exercise reverses aging in human skeletal muscle. PLoS ONE. 2(5): e465. Doi:10.1371/journal.pone.0000465

Morales, M.R., et al. (April 2012). Chronic conventional resistance exercise reduces blood pressure in stage 1 hypertensive men. *Journal of Strength and Conditioning Research*, 26(4): 1122-1129.

Kravitz, L. (2007). The 25 most significant health benefits of physical activity and exercise. *IDEA Fitness Journal*, 4(9): 54-63.

Kravitz, L. (1995). Exploring the mysteries of exercise. *IDEA Today*, 13(1): 48-55.

Scully, D. et al. (1998). Physical exercise and psychological well-being: A critical review. *British Journal of Sports and Medicine*, 32: 111-120.

Adverse effects of exercise in some individuals:

Bouchard, C. et al. (2012). Adverse metabolic response to regular exercise: Is it a rare or common occurrence? PLoS One. 7(5): e37887.doi: 10.1371/journal.pone.0037887

Fitness in general:

Dallbeck, L.C., & Kravitz, L. The history of fitness: From primitive to present times, how fitness has evolved and come of age. http://www.unm.edu/~lkravitz/Article%20folder/history.html

Harmon, K. (October 24, 2012). How slight sleep deprivation could add extra pounds. *Scientific American*: http://www. Scientificamerican.com/article.cfm?id=sleep-deprivation-obesity

Park, A., & Knauer, eds. (2008). Your body: A user's guide. *Time*. New York: Time Books.

Saadat, V. (June 16, 2011). The science behind exercise. *USCience Review*. University of Southern California: www-scf.usc.edu/~uscience/exercise_science.htm

U.S. News Health. The basics on fitness: Information on fitness.

http://www.health.usnews.com/health-conditions/heart-health/information-on-fitness

Fitness Statistics:

Centers for Disease Control and Prevention. NCHS data brief: Prevalence of obesity in the U.S., 2009-2010. Number 82, January 2012: http://www.cdc.gov/nchs/data/datbriefs/db82.htm

Centers for Disease Control and Prevention. State indicator report on physical activity, 2010. Atlanta, GA: U.S. Department of Human Services, 2010.

Centers for Disease Control and Prevention. U.S. physical activity statistics: www.cdc.gov/nccdphp/dnpa/physical/stats/index.htm

National Association for Sport and Physical Education & The American Heart Association. (2010). 2010 shape of the nation report: Status of physical education in the U.S.A. Reston, VA: National Association for Sport and Physical Education.

Prevalence of regular exercise within the general population:

Parker, S. (March 25, 2007). Physical fitness and exercise: the facts. *Health Guidance.* http://www.healthguidance.org/entry6299/1/Physical-Fitness-and-Exercise-The-Facts.html

Van Dusen, A. (February 27, 2008). Ten reasons you're a couch potato. Forbes.com. http://www.forbes.com/2008/02/27/health-couch-exercise-forbeslife-cx_avd_0227potato_print.html

Developing a fitness lifestyle:

Aldana, S. G. (2005). The culprit & the cure: Why lifestyle is the culprit behind America's poor health and how transforming that lifestyle is the cure. Mapleton, UT: Maple Mountain Press.

Fitness decline:

Too fat to fight: A report by Mission: Readiness. Military leaders for kids. http://www.MissionReadiness.org

Obesity problem:

F as in Fat: How obesity threatens America's future 2012. (September 2012). http://www.healthyamericans.org/report/100/

Kravitz, L. (2005). The growing problem of obesity. *IDEA Fitness Journal*, 2(10): 44-50.

Weight loss:

Stiegler, P. & Cunliffe, A. (2006). The role of diet and exercise for the maintenance of fat-free mass and resting metabolic rate during weight loss. *Sports Medicine*, 36(3): 239-262.

For a book that challenges many myths in the fitness world, see

Caulfield, T. (2013). The cure for everything: Untangling twisted messages about health, fitness, and happiness. Boston, MA: Beacon Press.

Chapter 2: Assessing Fitness

General issues related to the assessment of fitness:

Blair, S.N. & Church, T.S. (2004). The fitness, obesity, and health equation: Is physical activity the common denominator? *Journal of the American Medical Association*, 292(10): 1232-1234.

Germain, J.L. & Hausenblas, H.A. (2006). The relationship between perceived and actual physical fitness: A meta-analysis. *Journal of Applied Psychology*, 18(4): 283-96.

Skinner, J.S., Baldini, F.D., Gardner, A.W. & Gledhill, N. Exercise, fitness, and health: A consensus of current knowledge. Proceedings of the International Conference on Exercise, Fitness, and Health; May 29-June 3, 1988: pp. 109-126.

Thomas, J.R., Nelson, J.K. & Silverman, S.J. (2011). *Research methods in physical activity*, (6th ed.). Champaign, IL: Human Kinetics.

VO_2 Max (maximal oxygen consumption) is the gold standard in assessing aerobic fitness. It measures ventilation and oxygen and carbon dioxide of inhaled and exhaled air. I didn't include it in my measures because it can only be measured in a lab or facility equipped to monitor heart rate, arterial and venous oxygen content.

For a good read on heart health, including lipids, blood pressure, and other pertinent topics, see

Jaret, P. (2002) Heart healthy for life: The ultimate guide to preventing and reversing heart disease. Reader's Digest. Pleaseantville, NY: The Reader's Digest Association, Inc.

Heart.org. Understanding blood pressure readings. http://www.heart.org/HEARTORG/Conditions/HighBloodPressure/AboutHighBloodPressure

Mayo Clinic Staff. Triglycerides: Why do they matter? The Mayo Clinic. http://www. Mayoclinic.com/health/triglycerides/CL00015

Reference ranges for blood tests:

Wikipedia. Reference ranges for blood tests. en.wikipedia.org/wiki/Reference_ranges_for_blood_tests

Stats on the average male:

Elite Feet. Are you an average man? http://www.elitefeet.com/are-you-an-average-man.

Stats on common measures of health and fitness:

Mike, J.M. & Kravitz, L. (2010). Important risk factor and fitness assessment "numbers." *IDEA Fitness Journal*, 7(10): 22-27.

Kravitz, L. (2010). Waist-to-hip ratio, waist circumference and BMI. (2010). *IDEA Fitness Journal*, 7(9): 18-21.

Chapter 3: Aerobic Exercise

The Mayo Clinic Staff. Exercise for weight loss: Calories burned in 1 hour. The Mayo Clinic. http://www.mayoclinic.com/health/exercise/SM00109.

The merits of aerobic vs resistance exercise for the enhancement of fitness:

Kravitz, L. (1997). Aerobic exercise vs. resistance training: Is this the battle of the fitness titans. *IDEA Today*, 15(6): 52-58.

O'Toole, M.L. (1998). Overreaching and Overtraining in Endurance Athletes. In: Overtraining in Sport. Kreider, R.B., Fry, A.C., O'Toole, M.L. (Editors), Champaign: Human Kinetics.

Sprinting is better than long-distance running at promoting cardiovascular fitness:

Wiley, B. April 6, 2011). Better a sprint than a marathon: Brief intense exercise better than endurance training for preventing cardiovascular disease. *Science Daily*. Retrieved November 16, 2012, from http://www.sciencedaily.com/releases/2011/04/110405194101.htm

Dangers of extreme endurance exercise:

Park, A. (June 4, 2012). Extreme workouts: When exercise does more harm than good. *Time: Heartland*: http://heartland.time.com/2012/06/04/extreme-workouts-when-exercise-does-more-harm-than-good/

Exercise and the immune system:

Gleeson, M. (August 2007). Immune function in sport and exercise. *Journal of Applied Physiology*, 103(2): 693-699.

Koch, A. (2010). Immune response to exercise. *Brazilian Journal of Biomotricity*, 4(2): 92-103.

Riera, J. et al. (April 8, 2013). Dietary nucleotide improves markers of immune response to strenuous exercise under a cold environment. *Journal of International Society of Sports Nutrition,* 10(20): doi: 10.1186/1550-2783-10-20

Research on how aerobic exercise interferes with muscular hypertrophy:

Babcock, L., et al. (June 15, 2012). Concurrent aerobic exercise interferes with the satellite cell response to acute resistance exercise. *American Journal of Physiology*, 302(12): 458-65.

Bodine, S.C. et al. (November 2001). Akt/mTOR pathway is a crucial regulator of skeletal muscle hypertrophy and can prevent muscle atrophy in vivo. *Nature Cell Biology*, 3: 1014-19.

Nader, G.A. (2006). Concurrent strength and endurance training: From molecules to man. *Medical Science and Sports Exercise*, 38(11): 1965-70.

Wilson, J.M., et al. (August 26, 2012). Concurrent training: A meta-analysis examining interference of aerobic and resistance exercises. *Journal of Strength and Conditioning Research,* (8): 2293-307.

Calorie Burning:

Conn, C.A. & Kravitz, L. (2003). The remarkable calorie. *IDEA Personal Trainer*, 14(4): 28-35.

Fugelholm, M. & Kukkonen, H. (October 2000). Does physical activity prevent weight gain – a systematic review. *Obesity Reviews*, 1(2): 95-111.

Herrera, L, & Kravitz, l. (2009). Yes! You do burn fat during resistance exercise. *IDEA Fitness Journal*, 6(4): 17-19.

Kravitz, L. (2009). Calorie burning: It's time to think "outside the box:". *IDEA Fitness Journal*, 6(4): 32-38.

Ormsbee, M.J. et al. (2007). Fat metabolism and acute resistance exercise in trained men. *Journal of Applied Physiology*, 102: 1767-1772.

Chapter 4: The Science of Muscle

Research on muscular hypertrophy:

Ahtiainen, J.P. et al. (August 2005). Short vs long rest periods between sets in hypertrophic resistance training: Influence on muscle strength, size, and hormonal adaptations in trained men. *Journal of Strength & Conditioning Research*, 19(3).

Esgro, B. Super research feature: Maximizing skeletal muscle hypertrophy. DirectlyFitness.com

Hernandez, R.J. & Kravitz, L. (2003). The mystery of skeletal muscle hypertrophy. *ACSM's Health and Fitness Journal*, 7, 18-22.

Kwon, Y.S. & Kravitz, L. (2006). How do muscles grow? *IDEA Fitness Journal*, 3(2): 23-25.

Schoenfeld, B.J. (2010). The mechanisms of muscle hypertrophy and their application to resistance training. *Journal of Strength & Conditioning Research*, 24(10): 2857-72.

For a concise explanation of muscle growth, see:

Hamilton, D.L. & Barr, K. (2008). Muscle growth: No IGFs, ands or buts. *Journal of Physiology*, 586.1: 5-6.

Eccentric exercise, the lowering part of the movement, has been shown to do the most damage to muscle fibers and thus most likely contributes more to hypertrophy than the concentric part of the exercise.

Bubbico, A. & Kravitz, L. (2010). Eccentric exercise. IDEA Fitness Journal, 7(9): 50-59.

For a good book on hypertrophy training strategies, see

Hatfield, F. (1993). Hardcore bodybuilding: A scientific approach. McGraw-Hill, ISBN: 9780809237289.

Sarcopenia: Age-related muscle loss

Vella, C.A., & Kravitz, L. (2002). Sarcopenia: The mystery of muscle loss.

IDEA Personal Trainer, 13(4): 30-35.

Anabolic Steroids:

Roberts, A., & Clapp, B. (2005). Anabolic steroids: Ultimate research guide. Montgomery, TX: Anabolic Information, LLC.

Chapter 5: Approaches to Training

Brzycki, M., Ed. (2000). Maximize your training: Insights from leading strength and fitness professionals. Chicago, IL: Masters Press. (**This book covers many questions and issues related to various training approaches.**)

Bushman, B.A. (2011). ACSM's complete guide to fitness and health. Champaign, IL: Human Kinetics.

Corbin, C.B. (2004). Concepts of physical fitness: Active lifestyles for wellness (12th ed.). McGraw Hill, ISBN: 9780072843743.

Hoeger, W. & Hoeger, S. (2009). Lifetime physical fitness and wellness: A personalized program (10th ed.). Belmont, CA: Wadsworth, Cengage Learning.

For more information on Crossfit, see the following:

Glassman, G. (April 2007). Understanding crossfit. *Crossfit Journal*, Issue 56. www.crossfit.com

Crossfit Foundations: Forging elite fitness. www.crossfit.com

What is fitness? (October 2002). Crossfit Journal. www.crossfit.com

A review of crossfit: http://www.sweatpit.com/forum/ubbthreads.php

Chapter 6: Building Muscle

Training protocols for optimal gains in muscle:

Brzycki, M., Ed. (2000). Maximize your training: Insights from leading strength and fitness professionals. Chicago, IL: Masters Press. (This book covers many questions and issues related to different training approaches.)

Kravitz, L. (2007). Training to failure. *IDEA Fitness Journal*, 4(9): 23-24.

Amount of training volume for optimal muscular hypertrophy:

Krieger, J.W. (2010). Single vs. multiple sets of resistance exercise for muscle hypertrophy: a meta-analysis. *Journal of Strength & Conditioning Research*, 24(4): 1150-59.

Braith, R.W., Graves, J.E., Pollock, M.L., Leggett, S.L., Carpenter, D.M., & Colvin, A.B. (1989). Comparison of 2 vs 3 days/week of variable resistance training during 10- and 18-week programs. *International Journal of Sports Medicine*, 10(6): 450-54.

Rhea, M.R., Alvar, B.A., Burkett, L.N., & Ball, S.D. (2003). A meta-analysis to determine the dose response for strength development. *Medical Science and Sports Exercise*, 35(3): 456-64.

Wolfe, B.L., LeMura, L.M., & Cole, P.J. (2004). Quantitative analysis of single- vs. multiple-set programs in resistance training. *Journal of Strength & Conditioning Research*, 18(1): 35-47.

Optimal duration of rest periods: The following studies found no significant differences in muscular hypertrophy using 2- or 4-minute rest periods between sets.

Ahtiainen, J.P. et al. (August 2005). Short vs long rest periods between sets in hypertrophic resistance training: Influence on muscle strength, size, and hormonal adaptations in trained men. *Journal of Strength & Conditioning Research*, 19(3): 572-582.

Willardson, J.M., & Burkett, L.N. (2008). The effect of different rest intervals between sets on volume components and strength gains. *Journal of Strength & Conditioning Research*, 22(1): 146-52.

Information on various hypertrophy and strength routines:

Matthews, M. (2012). Bigger, Leaner, Stronger: The simple science of building the ultimate male body (Kindle version). Waterbury Publishers.

Stoppani, J. (2011). Encyclopedia of muscle & strength. Human Kinetics.

For a good book on hypertrophy training strategies, see

Hatfield, F. (1993). Hardcore bodybuilding: A scientific approach. McGraw-Hill, ISBN: 9780809237289.

For a good review of overtraining, see

Halson, S.L. & Jeukendrup, A.E. (2004). Does overtraining exist? An analysis of overreaching and overtraining research. *Sports Medicine*, 34(14): 967-981.

The effects of some trendy training modalities:

Binnie, M.J., Dawson, B., Pennington, H., Landers, G. & Peeling, P. (April 2013). Effect of training surface on acute physiological responses after interval training. *Journal of Strength and Conditioning Research*, 27(4): 1047-1056.

Chapter 7: Training Myths

Bee, P. (June 4, 2007). The fitness myths. *The Guardian*: http://www.guardian.co.uk/lifeandstyle/2007/ju

Caulfield, T. (2013). The cure for everything: Untangling twisted messages about health, fitness, and happiness. Boston, MA: Beacon Press.

FitnessMagazine.com. The top 10 fitness myths you're probably wrong about. http://www.fitnessmagazine.com/fitness

Graves, G. (June 6, 2008). Forget fad diets: Get the facts on weight loss. *NBC News: Diet and Nutrition*: http://www.msnbc.msn.com/id/24843493/ns/health-diet

Haddad, M. et al. (2013). Static stretching can impair explosive performance for at least 24 hours. *Journal of Strength Conditioning Research*, 27: 973-77.

Matthews, M. (2012). Muscle Myths: 50 health & fitness mistakes you don't know you're making. Waterbury Publishers, ISBN: 147514377X.

Chapter 8: Ongoing Debates

Gannelli, S. (2000). Free weights versus machines, In: Maximize your training: Insights from leading strength and fitness professionals, Matt Brzycki, Ed. Chicago, IL: Masters Press.

Brzycki, M., Ed. (2000). Maximize your training: Insights from leading strength and fitness professionals. Chicago, IL: Masters Press. (This book covers many questions and issues related to different training approaches.)

Buchan, D.S. et al. (2011). The effects of time and intensity of exercise on novel and established markers of cardiovascular disease in adolescent youth. *American Journal of Human Biology*, doi: 10.1002/ajhb.21166

Nelson, J. & Kravitz, L. (2002). Super slow resistance training. *IDEA Personal Trainer,* 13(6): 13-15.

Wiley, B. April 6, 2011). Better a sprint than a marathon: Brief intense exercise better than endurance training for preventing cardiovascular disease. *Science Daily*. Retrieved November 16, 2012, from http://www.sciencedaily.com/releases/2011/04/110405194101.htm

Periodization:

Fleck, S.J. (1999). Periodized strength training: A critical review. *Journal of Strength and Conditioning Research*, 13: 82-89.

Frankel, C.C., & Kravitz, L. (2000). Periodization. *IDEA Personal Trainer*, 11 (1): 15-16.

Making workload alterations (8RM, 6RM, 4RM) every workout was more effective in eliciting strength gains than doing so every 4 weeks. This finding supports my contention that traditional periodization is less effective at enhancing hypertrophy than making sufficient workload variations within each workout.

Rhea, M.R., Ball, S.D., Phillips, W.T., & Burkett, L.N. (2002). A comparison of linear and daily undulating periodized programs with equated volume and intensity for strength. *Journal of Strength & Conditioning Research,* 16(2): 250-55.

Chapter 9: Fitness Fads

Daoust, P. (January 7, 2011). A history of fitness fads. *The Guardian*. Online: http://www.guardian.co.uk/lifeand style/2011/jan/08/history-fitness-fads

The 25 biggest fitness fads of all time: The most laughable and most functional fitness fads. *Men's Fitness*. Online: http://www.mensfitness.com/gear/fashion-and-trends/the-25-biggest-fitness-fads-of-all-time

Trendy diets:

Agatston, A. (2005). The South Beach diet: The delicious, doctor-designed, foolproof plan for fast and healthy weight loss. St. Martin's Griffin, ISBN: 9780312315214.

Atkins, R. (1981). Dr. Atkins' diet revolution. Bantam, ISBN: 9780553271577.

Cordain, L. (2010). The Paleo diet revised: Lose weight and get healthy by eating the foods you were designed to eat. Houghton Mifflin Harcourt, ISBN: 9780470913024.

Dukan, P. (2011). The Dukan diet: 2 steps to lose the weight, 2 steps to keep it off forever. Harmony, ISBN: 9780307887962.

Eades, M.R. & Eades, M.D. (1999). Protein Power: The high-protein/low-carbohydrate way to lose weight, feel fit, and boost your health – in just weeks! Bantam, ISBN: 9780553380781.

Gallop, R. (2010). The G.I. diet. Workman, ISBN: 9780761144793.

Katahn, M. (1989). The T-factor diet. W.W. Norton & Company, ISBN: 9780393321432.

Ornish, D. (2000). Eat more, weigh less: Dr. Dean Ornish's life choice program for losing weight safely while eating abundantly. William Morrow Paperbacks, ISBN: 9780060959579.

Pritikin, R. (2000). The Pritikin principle: The calorie density solution. Time Life Education, ISBN: 9780737016161.

Sears, B. & Lawren, B. (1995). Enter the zone: A dietary road map. Regan Book, ISBN: 9780060391508.

Whitney, D. & Whitney, C. (1997). Eat right 4 your type: The individualized diet solution to staying healthy, living longer, & achieving your ideal weight. Putnam Adult, ISBN: 9780399142550.

Chapter 10: Nutrition Basics

General Nutrition:

Cataldo, C.B., DeBruyne, L.K., & Whitney, E.N. (1995). Nutrition & diet therapy: Principles and practice, (4th ed.). Minneapolis/St. Paul: West Publishing Company.

Golomb, B.A., Koperski, S., et al. (March 2012). Chocolate at breakfast: Association between more frequent chocolate consumption and lower body mass index. *Archives of Internal Medicine*, 172: 519-21.

Gorman, C. (October 20, 2003). How to eat smarter. [Health Feature] *Time.*

Macronutrient Ratios:

Bravata DM, Sanders L, Huang J, Krumholz HM, Olkin I, Gardner CD, Bravata DM (2003). Efficacy and safety of low-carbohydrate diets: a systematic review. *Journal of the American Medical Association*, 9;289(14):1837-50.

Grundy, S.M. (1999). The optimal ratio of fat to carbohydrate in the diet. *Annual Review of Nutrition*, 19: 325-41.

Krieger JW, Sitren HS, Daniels MJ, Langkamp-Henken B (2006). Effects of variation in protein and carbohydrate intake on body mass and composition during energy restriction: a meta-regression 1. *American Journal of Clinical Nutrition,* 83(2): 260-74.

The Glycemic Index:

Mayo, J.J. & Kravitz, L. (2009). Glycemic index: Weight loss sham or sensation. *IDEA Fitness Journal*, 6(1): 15-17.

Evaluation of low-carb diets:

Very Low Carbohydrate diets have been shown to be more effective for short-term weight loss (less than 6 months to 1 year) than calorie restrictive diet and/or low fat diets. Improvements in blood pressure, lipids, fasting glucose, and insulin were also observed.

Brehm, B.J., Seeley, R.J., Daniels, S.R., & D'Alessio, D.A. (2003). A randomized trial comparing a very low carbohydrate diet and a calorie-restricted low fat diet on body weight and cardiovascular risk factors in healthy women. *Journal of Clinical Endocrinology Metabolism*, 88(4):1617-23.

Foster GD, Wyatt HR, Hill JO, McGuckin BG, Brill C, Mohammed BS, Szapary PO, Rader DJ, Edman JS, Klein S (May 22, 2003). A randomized trial of a low-carbohydrate diet for obesity. *New England Journal of Medicine,* 348(21):2082-90.

Samaha FF, Iqbal N, Seshadri P, Chicano KL, Daily DA, McGrory J, Williams T, Williams M, Gracely EJ, Stern L (2003). A low-carbohydrate as compared with a low-fat diet in severe obesity. *New England Journal of Medicine,* 348(21): 2074-81.

Johnston et al 2006 found that a ketogenic low-carbohydrate diet (beginning with ~5% carbohydrate, 60% fat) and nonketogenic low-carbohydrate diet (40% carbohydrate, 30% fat) were equally effective in reducing body weight and insulin resistance. However, ketogenic group experienced several adverse metabolic and emotional effects such as higher inflammatory risk (arachidonic acid:eicosapentaenoic acid ratios in plasma phospholipids) and lower perceptions vigor. (Source):http://www.exrx.net/FatLoss/MacronutrientRatio.html

Johnston CS, Tjonn SL, Swan PD, White A, Hutchins H, & Sears B (2006). Ketogenic low-carbohydrate diets have no metabolic advantage over nonketogenic low-carbohydrate diets. *American Society for Clinical Nutrition,* 83(5): 1055-1061.

Protein Requirements:

Bilsborough, S. & Mann, N. (April 16, 2006). A review of issues of dietary protein intake in humans. *International Journal of Sports Nutrition, Exercise, and Metabolism*, 16(2): 129-52.

Bosse, J.D. & Dixon, B.M. (September 8, 2012). Dietary protein to maximize resistance training: A review and examination of protein spread and change theories. *Journal of the International Society of Sports Nutrition*, 9:42.

Layman, D.K. (March 13, 2009). Dietary guidelines should reflect new understandings about adult protein needs, *Nutrition & Metabolism*, 6:12.

Tarnopolsky, M.A. et al. (November 1, 1992). Evaluation of protein requirements for trained strength athletes. *Journal of Applied Physiology*, 73(5): 1986-95.

Nutrient Timing: The idea that when you eat, especially in regard to pre- and post-training, enhances muscular hypertrophy or general fitness. The following study casts doubt on this idea.

Aragon, A.A. & Schoenfeld, B.J. (January 29, 2013). Nutrient timing revisited: Is there a post-exercise anabolic window? *Journal of International Society of Sports Nutrition*, 10:5.

Chambers, A. & Kravitz, L. (2009). Nutrient timing: The new frontier in fitness performance. *AKWA: The Official Publication of the Aquatic Exercise Association,* 22(4): 4-6.

Chruchward-Venne, T.A., Burd, N.A., & Phillips, S.M. (2012). Nutritional regulation of muscle protein synthesis with resistance exercise: strategies to enhance anabolism. *Nutrition and Metabolism*, 9:40: doi: 10.1186/1743-7075-9-40

Stark, M., Lukaszuk, J., Prawitz, A. & Salacinski, A. (2012). Protein timing and its effects on muscular hypertrophy and strength in individuals engaged in weight training. *Journal of the International Society of Sports Nutrition*, 9(54).

Diet and nutrition myths:

Fit Facts: Diet myths debunked. (2009). *American Council on Exercise*: http://www.acefitness.org/fitfacts/pdfs/fitfacts/

Graves, G. (June 6, 2008). Forget fad diets: Get the facts on weight loss. *NBC News: Diet and Nutrition*: http://www.msnbc.msn.com/id/24843493/ns/health-diet

Kravitz, L. (2011) Metabolism make-over: Fact or fiction? *IDEA Fitness Journal*, 8(6): 21-23.

Training in a fed or fasting state:

Paoli, A., Marcolin, G., Zonin, F., Neri, M., Sivieri, A., & Pacelli, Q. (2011). Exercising fasting or fed to enhance fat loss? Influence of food intake on respiratory ratio and excess postexercise oxygen consumption after a bout of endurance training. *International Journal of Sport Nutrition and Exercise Metabolism*, 21: 48-54.

Meal Frequency – 3 meals a day may do a better job of controlling hunger than multiple feedings.

Leidy, H. & Campbell, W. (December 1, 2010). The effect of eating frequency on appetite control and food intake: Brief synopsis of controlled feeding studies. The Journal of Nutrition, Online, doi: 10.3945/jn.109.114389

Ohkawara, K., Cornier, M.A., Kohrt, W.M., & Melanson, E.L. (February 2013). Effects of increased meal frequency on fat oxidation and perceived hunger. *Obesity (Silver Spring)*, 21(2): 336-43.

Supplementation:

Beta Alanine. Wikipedia.com
Creatine. Wikipedia.com

Derave, W. et al. (August 9, 2009). Beta-Alanine supplementation augments muscle carnosine content and attenuates fatigue during repeated isokinetic contraction bouts in trained sprinters. *Journal of Applied Physiology*, 103 (5): 1736.

Kern, B., & Robinson, T. (July 31, 2009). Effects of beta-alanine supplementation on performance and body composition in collegiate wrestlers and American football players. *Journal of the International Society of Sports Nutrition,* 6, (supplement 1) p.2.

Terjung, R.L. (2000). American College of Sports Medicine roundtable: The physiological and health effects of oral creatine supplementation. *Medicine and Science in Sports and Exercise*, 32(3): 706-717.

Volek, J.S. etal. (1999). Performance and muscle fiber adaptations to creatine supplementation and heavy resistance training. *Medical Science, Sports, and Exercise*, 31(8): 1147-1156.

MSN Health. (October 6, 2000). What you should know about dietary supplements. http://content.health.msn.com/content/article/1671.50959

Obesity Myths:

Casazza, K. et al. (January 31, 2013). Myths, presumptions, and facts about obesity. *New England Journal of Medicine*, 368: 446-454.

Weight loss:

Parker-Pope, T. (December 28, 2011). The fat trap. *The New York Times Magazine*: www.nytimes.com/2012/01/01/magazine/tara-parker-pope-fat-trap.html

Kruger, J., Blanck, H.M. & Gillespie, C. (2006). Dietary and physical activity behaviors among adults successful at weight loss maintenance. International *Journal of Behavioral Nutrition and Physical Activity*, 3(17): doi: 10.1186/1479-5868-3-17

Stiegler, P. & Cunliffe, A. (2006). The role of diet and exercise for the maintenance of fat-free mass and resting metabolic rate during weight loss. *Sports Medicine*, 36(3): 239-262.

Chapter 11: The Dark Side of Fitness

Bamber, D., Cockerill, I. & Carroll, D. (2000). The pathological status of exercise dependence. *British Journal of Sports Medicine*, 34: 125-132.

Davis, C. & Woodside, D. (May 2002). Sensitivity to the rewarding effects of food and exercise in the eating disorders. *Comprehensive Psychiatry*, 43(3): 189-194.

Dess, N.K. (May/June 2000). Killer workout: The dark side of diet and exercise. *Psychology Today*, p.26.

Hurst, R., Hale, B., Smith, D. & Collins, A. (2000). Exercise dependence, social physique anxiety, and social support in experienced and inexperienced bodybuilders and weightlifters. *British Journal of Sports Medicine*, 34: 431-435.

Morrisette, N. & Kravitz, L. (2006). Exercise addiction. *IDEA Fitness Journal*, 3(5): 20-23.

Szabo, A. (1995). The impact of exercise deprivation on well-being of habitual exercisers. *Australian Journal of Science and Medicine in Sport*, 27(3): 68-75.

Chapter 12: Mind Over Muscle

For more on the mental aspect of training and sports see:

Bauman, J. (May/June 2000). The gold medal. *Psychology Today*, p. 62-68.

Orlick, T. (2000). In pursuit of excellence: How to win in sport and life through mental training (3rd ed.). Human Kinetics.

Developing good habits:

Heitler, S. (February 29, 2012). Changing habits beats reliance on willpower. Psychology Today. Online: http://www.psychologytoday.com

Exercise and metal health:

Colcombe, S. & Kramer, A. (March 2003). Fitness effects on the cognitive function of older adults: A meta-analytic study. *Psychological Science*, 14(2): 125-30.

Kravitz, L. (2010). Exercise and the brain: It will make you want to work out. *IDEA Fitness Journal*, 7(2): 18-19.

O'Connor, P.J., Herring, M.P. and Carvalho, A. (2010). Mental health benefits of strength training in adults. *American Journal of Lifestyle Medicine,* 4(5): 377-396.

Ramirez, A. & Kravitz, L. (2012). Resistance training improves mental health. *IDEA Fitness Journal*, 9(1): 20-22.

Scully, D. et al. (1998). Physical exercise and psychological well-being: A critical review. *British Journal of Sports and Medicine*, 32: 111-120.

For more on the concept of flow see:

Csikszentmihalyi, M. (1990). *Flow: The psychology of optimal experience*, New York: Harper & Row.

Jackson, S., & Csikszentmihalyi, M. (1999). *Flow in sports*. Human Kinetics.

Epilogue

The case for small changes adding up over time:

Kravitz, L. (2010). Small changes and the obesity epidemic. *IDEA Fitness Journal*, 7(1): 18-20.

Excellent sources concerning recommendations for promoting fitness within the general population:

National Center for Health Statistics. (2010). Healthy people 2010: Final review. Hyattville, MD: www.cdc.gov/nchs/data/hpdata2010/hp2010_final_review.pdf

U.S. Department of Health and Human Services. The Surgeon General's vision for a healthy and fit nation. Rockville, MD: U.S. Department of Health and Human Services, Office of the Surgeon General, January 2010: http://www.surgeongeneral.gov/initiatives/healthy-fit-nation/obesityvision2010.pdf

White House Task Force on Childhood Obesity: Report to the President. Solving the problem of childhood obesity within a generation: www.letsmove.gov/sites/letsmove.gov/files/taskforce_on_Childhood_Obesity_May2010_FullReport.pdf